Holistic Aromatherapy Comprehensive Guide

JennScents®, Inc.
Clermont, Florida, USA

JennScents®

Holistic Aromatherapy Comprehensive Guide

A Compilation of JennScents® Holistic Aromatherapy Education, Research & Recipes

Written By:

Jennifer Pressimone

Holistic Aromatherapist, Herbalist & Aromatherapy Evangelist

www.JennScents.com | www.JennScentsInstitute.com

JennScents® Holistic Aromatherapy Comprehensive Guide
By: Jennifer Pressimone

ISBN 978-0-9971463-0-1

Published by JennScents, Inc., Clermont, Florida
Printed in the United States of America
First Printing 2015

Book Layout: Jennifer Pressimone

Cover Design: Jennifer Pressimone, Earl "Bud" Peck, Jr. & J. Maureen Henderson

Editor & Proofreader: Kimberly McCormick

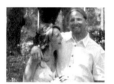

Dedicated to my husband Steve, for allowing me to pursue my dreams with
full support and encouragement; to my parents for their never-ending support;
and to my many, brilliant aromatherapy mentors.

In memory of
my grandfather, James Fred Stewart
and
my father, Richard Allan Hoshell

Acknowledgements

This comprehensive guide was a decade in the making. It is a compilation of education, observations, trial and error that I have personally experienced during my holistic health journey to date. I am a firm believer in paying forward the gifts that have been presented to us, so other lives may be enriched and inspired.

This book is for my family, friends, clients and aromatherapy lovers everywhere.

First and foremost, I'd like to give special thanks to my family, without them, none of my existence would be possible. They have been my strength, my guidance, my supporters and my inspiration. To my husband, Steve, who continues to be my rock each and every day. To my parents for their endless support and for always making things happen behind the scenes. To my siblings, nieces, nephews and cousins…we are family strong!

To my friends, who have watched me grow, thrive and evolve over the years and have allowed me to touch their lives, as they have touched mine.

To my clients for giving me such challenging cases to learn from, allowing me to be the best I can be.

To aromatherapy lovers everywhere, thank you for loving aromatherapy as much as I do and for seeing it for its fullest potential and power. It is a gift we must hold sacred and respect on all levels.

A special thank you to my many, amazing, brilliant and extraordinary mentors and educators I've been blessed to cross paths with. You have helped shape my knowledge, sharpen my skills, recognize my gifts and unite our community. You have turned my journey into meaning, and I am honored to call you my friend.

J. Maureen Henderson, the best friend, mentor and big sister a person could ask for. She encouraged me to investigate the world of holistic health, and look what happened…JennScents was born.

Dr. Bruce Berkowsky, one of the best mentors a person could ask for. He is such an incredible human being, full of significant, thought-provoking, inspiring and profound knowledge, wisdom and philosophy. He continues to inspire me to be my best, each and every moment, being true to my authentic self.

Wendimere Reilly, words are not enough to describe my fondness and deep appreciation. A true best friend, wonderful human being, inspiration and one my biggest cheerleaders. Wendimere first introduced me to the word and art of aromatherapy. She empowered me to take control of my own health. She helped me conquer my fear of public speaking, even after I passed out practicing in front of my own mom. She helped me find my confidence and purpose while supporting my aromatherapy and life journey. To her, I am eternally grateful.

Cheryl Ralph, a life-changing friend and teacher who endured some of my roughest times with me, helping me find the silver lining in each and every situation. I also have to thank Chrystina Katz for introducing us and being a part of our intense, intentional, purpose-filled sisterhood. They both ignited my power and strength to create this book.

Dr. Kimberly Balas, an amazing person and friend with one of the most brilliant minds and personalities on the planet. Not only can I say I know a rocket scientist, but I can say she truly saved my life. I exist and am able to share my wisdom because of her. She was the first to inspire me to pursue authentic mind-body health, connecting the emotions to the physical body for true optimum healing.

Larissa Jones is a kind and loving person who showed me the softer side of aromatherapy. She gave me structure and confidence to begin teaching my skills and insight.

Steven Horne, a gifted teacher who taught me the basics to advanced level natural health fundamentals. He is selfless when it comes to sharing his wisdom.

Denise Sherman, my very first formal aromatherapy teacher. She gave me a solid foundation in understanding aromatherapy, respecting it and employing it for mind-body health.

Gabriel Mojay, a brilliant human being and teacher. He taught me how to be passionate and intentional with aromatherapy, and elevated my skills to a whole new level, allowing me tap into a deeper part of my soul.

Dr. Jay Vanden Heuval, one of the most enthusiastic educators, practitioners and colleagues I know. He has taught me so many natural health nuggets and knowledge over the years, helping me help myself and so many others. He has played a part in helping me tap into my inner soul gifts.

Jeanne Rose, taught me core fundamentals of aromatherapy. I first visited her at a seminar in Fort Lauderdale in 2003. She was an inspiration and role model to be a true, professional aromatherapist.

Sylla Sheppard-Hanger, taught me how to be resilient in the ever-changing aromatherapy realm, and to be true to myself, with an open heart.

Ken Rose, who helped me bring all of my books from formatting to print.

And to the countless other mentors, teachers, friends and colleagues not named, Thank you!

A Special Note From The Author to the Reader

There are numerous books on aromatherapy to choose from, so why did I feel compelled to write this book? Well, as with everything we all experience in life, our own personal view may be different than someone else's. We have different insight and perspective. We may have picked up on some different skills to solve a particular problem. I have personally experienced a great deal of challenges, struggles and successes in life. My mom instilled in me when I was young, to always pay forward the blessings brought forth to me, enriching another's life.

My hope for you, the reader, is to gain a greater foundation in aromatherapy with reference to science and evidence of its efficacy; to immerse yourself in the core principles of aromatherapy so that you can develop your own skills and blending techniques to pay it forward, and help others; and to provoke thought and inspire new dialogue in the aromatherapy realm. This continuum of giving with reciprocal receiving can spread far and wide across the globe. You will benefit from the lessons I have learned along the way. Gain knowledge about the helpful essential oils I have found for a plethora of physical, mental and emotional health concerns. There is information for the beginner just starting out, to the advanced, professional aromatherapists. I hope this will become a staple in your repertory of reference books.

About The Author

Jennifer Pressimone is a holistic aromatherapist, herbalist, author, international educator and Teaching Diplomate of Spiritual PhytoEssencing. She owns JennScents, Inc. and JennScents Institute. JennScents, Inc. is a holistic aromatherapy business, creating therapeutic products to meet client needs. The JennScents Institute offers a holistic aromatherapy certification program, NAHA Level I & II and NCBTMB approved.

Jennifer was first introduced to holistic health in the late 1990's during her battle with Crohn's, colitis and IBS. She integrated herbal and aromatic remedies with conventional medicine to facilitate in her recovery from the devastation her body, and mind endured. She first learned about the importance of probiotics and enzymes, and the power of essential oils. The very first essential oil she smelled was Roman Chamomile. How fitting, as chamomile is a caretaker, nurturer and incredible anti-inflammatory and antispasmodic oil. Her friend, Wendimere Reilly invited her to a tea n' chat event where she shared the benefits of chamomile, and made up a roll-on for Jennifer to try for her intestinal spasms and frail body. Guess what, Jennifer tried the roll-on that night and had results in in just 10 minutes. Her intestinal cramps subsided, her mind calmed down and she could breathe, tension free for the first time in years. Needless to say, she was hooked on aromatherapy ever since.

Jennifer started JennScents, Inc. in 2002 after a career in banking and insurance. Her family owned business is dedicated to providing superior quality aromatherapy products and holistic education. Her holistic approach is aimed to help others help themselves through empowerment and knowledge, assisting in the decision making process of their health with genuine wisdom, education and high quality products.

Jennifer now considers herself to be an Aromatherapy Evangelist, meaning she is an enthusiastic advocate for promoting and empowering others with authentic aromatherapy wisdom to inspire physical, mental, emotional and spiritual health. She is dedicated to bringing greater awareness to the use and benefits of true aromatherapy, helping people and pets achieve emotional and physical well-being, holistically. Through her institute and research, she pledges to make significant contributions to the world of aromatherapy and empower others to help themselves. Jennifer is passionate about her family, pets, friends, aromatherapy and spending time in nature.

Jennifer is a graduate of the University of Central Florida with a Bachelor of Arts Degree in Psychology and Teacher Diplomate in Spiritual PhytoEssencing (deep emotional healing) from Dr. Bruce Berkowsky. She is a professional member, Regional Director and Vice President with NAHA, the National Association of Holistic Aromatherapy.

Contents

Introduction

Aromatherapy is a practice that has been utilized for over 9000 years. From our ancestors to our great grandparents to our current generation, aromatherapy continues to flourish and offer therapeutic properties to our everyday lives. In fact, France physicians prescribe essential oils on a regular basis to address physical and emotional concerns, as does many other European and Asian countries.

In the United States, aromatherapy has become a household name in personal care and household products such as bath and body washes, skin and care, cleaning supplies and in food dishes. It is a staple in almost every hotel to have aromatherapy-based bath and shower products. Almost every retailer in the US, and abroad sell some form of aromatherapy-based products. Not only do they make us smell good, but they also help us feel better. The health benefits of aromatherapy are being scientifically proven more today than ever before. From its antioxidant properties, to anti-inflammatory, antispasmodic, antiviral and the list goes on. It is also becoming a hot commodity in real estate, home architecture (ventilation and shower systems) and technology (diffusers for the home, car, computers and movie theaters).

Scientific studies conducted have paved the way for grant monies to be awarded to health care facilities for continued support in helping persons with various mental health challenges such as Alzheimer's, Parkinson's and Dementia. Other grants have been awarded to help minimize negative effects such as nausea when receiving chemotherapy and radiation (Children's Hospital, Los Angeles, 2013). The Nobel Prize in Physiology or Medicine in 2004 was awarded to two American scientists, Richard Axel, MD and Linda Buck, Ph.D., who won for their discoveries of odorant receptors and the organization of the olfactory system.

Aromatherapy is not only being employed in wellness and health care facilities, but car manufacturers are now joining in on the action. The 2014 Mercedes Benz S-Class sedans came with a $350 option of a built-in fragrance atomizer system and four exclusive custom cologne scents. The system, located in the glove compartment, offered an "active perfuming system" dispersed via the A/C vents and controlled by the driver *(http://mazurgroupla.com/scent-with-intent-growing-demand-for-non-traditional-uses-of-aromatherapy/)*.

These generational advances have helped aromatherapy become one of the hottest and fastest growing segments in the natural health business arena. According to IBISWorld in January 2015, they estimate the essential oil manufacturing industry is growing faster than the overall economy. They anticipate for 2010-2020, the industry's contribution to the economy is expected to grow an average of 2.8% annually, compared to US GDP (growth domestic product) average of 2.5% over the same period *(http://www.ibisworld.com/industry/essential-oil-manufacturing.html)*. Wellness has become more of a way of life for millions of people, rather than just a "fad". If you look at some of the top global wellness trends for 2015, they include workplace wellness programs, wellness communities and programs, wellness spa treatments, aromatherapy driven products and health protocols *(http://www.spafinder.com/content/2015-global-spa-wellness-trends)*.

Unfortunately, there is much misinformation in our society about the true and holistic benefits of using 100% pure and authentic essential oils versus fragrant oils and synthetic scents. It is a mission of mine and the intent of this comprehensive guide to educate you not only about the genuine benefits and uses of essential oils but how to apply them to your everyday life and routines. This guide offers simple, effective and easy to make recipes for a variety of common health concerns, as well as foundational knowledge and science to explain how and why aromatherapy works.

"Scents create memories that last a lifetime and remind us to be us." Jennifer Pressimone

History

Past

Aromatherapy is a practice that has been around for thousands of years. It has played a profound part of every culture at some point in time…Egyptian, Greek, Roman, Chinese, Indian, Persian, Native American and many others. It is said to have originated with the Egyptians. They made numerous aromatic perfumes for specific events and rituals, used for skin care preparations and certain scents such as cinnamon and frankincense were employed in their mummification process. In fact, the essential oils proved to be so powerful that the fragrance of frankincense and rosewood could still be smelled when King Tut's tomb was opened in 1922. Egyptians have been noted to be involved in the advancement of distilling essential oils, however, it was Avicenna, a Persian philosopher and scientist that was credited with the development and production of the distillation process. He along with many others from then until now, have perfected the equipment and methods.

The Greek and Romans made many contributions to the aromatic world. The Greeks laid mint leaves on the floors of temples and the Romans wore "laurels" on their head with bay fragrances (hence bay laurel), mint and rosemary to commemorate special occasions and victories in battle. Ancient Greek and Roman physicians used aromatherapy to treat a variety of health concerns such as headaches, respiratory and urinary distresses. Hippocrates, known as the Father of Medicine, learned many herbal and aromatic therapies. He recommended taking a daily aromatic bath and massage to prolong life.

Ayurveda, meaning "the science of life" is a one of the oldest natural health systems that was, and still is, used for cultural ceremonies and rituals, health care and perfumes. It was used by many physicians in conjunction with other therapeutic remedies for prevention, restoration and harmonization of all three doshas, or impurities, which are vata, pitta and kapha. These are responsible for balancing environment, body, mind and spirit, simultaneously.

Traditional Chinese Medicine (TCM), as well as Tibetan medicine, both have roots in Ayurveda. Like many other cultures, they incorporated aromatherapy into their medical practices, massage therapy, healing baths, acupuncture, religious ceremonies and food dishes to bring harmony and vitality to our "chi", also known in Western culture as life energy or vital force. Their goal is for balanced mind and body coexistence.

In the 17th century, the Black Plague ravished Europe killing more than one third of the population. Commoners and doctors used walking sticks with hollow tops filled with aromatics (essential oils) and herbs to ward off the plague. They would burn piles of herbs and aromatics in the streets to rid the horrid smell that emanated from the plagued bodies. During the French plague to avoid contracting the disease, doctors covered themselves from head to toe in leather and beaked masks filled with aromatic herbs (this is where the term "Quack" was said to have originated). Others who were immune from the plague included glove makers who dipped newly made gloves in essential oils; perfumers who at that time used only 100% pure, unadulterated essential oils; and thieves who stole the jewels and treasures from plagued bodies to give to the king.

The bible has over 100 references to herbs and essential oils. Perhaps one of the most famous stories was the Gifts of the Magi to Baby Jesus. These gifts were frankincense, myrrh and gold. The frankincense and myrrh, as well as other essential oils, were more prized than the gold. Also, Mary Magdalene anointed Jesus' feet with spikenard after washing them and drying them with her hair *(John 12:3)*.

A popular name in the aromatherapy arena is René-Maurice Gattefossé (1881-1950). He was a French chemist and pioneer who is credited with coining the term "aromatherapy" and wrote *Gattefosse's Aromatherapies*, the first book about aromatherapy, which was translated from French to English in 1937. Gattefossé came from a family in the French perfume trade and made many discoveries and advancements throughout his years, before passing in 1950. One of his most popular findings was the power of lavender for wound healing, after he was badly burned in a laboratory explosion *(http://roberttisserand.com/2011/04/gattefosses-burn/)*.

Gattefossé may have introduced aromatherapy to the world of science but it was Dr. Jean Valnet (1920-1995), a French aromatherapist, psychiatrist, military and civilian physician and surgeon, who is most recognized for bringing notoriety and popularity to the field of aromatherapy integration and aromatic medicine. He used aromatherapy applications during World War II to treat battle wounds and later to wean patients off chemical medicines.

Present

Today, aromatherapy is a significant tool many people use for relaxation, invigoration and to promote an overall good, happy feeling. Many commercial businesses, are incorporating aromatic scents into their body, skin, hair and cleaning products. A health care facility in Texas was recognized for successfully incorporating aromatherapy practices into their facilities and aiding illnesses such as cancer and Alzheimer's disease. Aromatherapy is even making its way into night clubs, zoos, and computer occupations.

In the modern development of aromatherapy, we are seeing scent driven cleaning products, bath and body products, food dishes and nursing home, hospice and hospital protocols. For example, Hospice of Florida Suncoast has integrated essential oil use in palliative care via massage, aromatic mist (such as a bereavement blend) and diffusion.

We are not only seeing aromatherapy being employed for fun as with bubble baths and candles, but we are seeing an increase in health restoration practices. Organic Style Magazine in June 2005 shared that pink grapefruit essential oil helped curb appetite and sweet cravings according to research by Institute of Aromatherapy in Toronto. Other studies showed angelica, black pepper, peppermint and bergamot helped with smoking addictions. Rose placed on the upper lip helped decrease depression.

A January 2010 study published at www.PubMed.com found that not only does the smell of jasmine create a sense of alertness, it can also serve as a way to help with depressive thoughts. Researchers found that the stimulating effect of jasmine oil can aid in the relief of depression and lead to an uplifted mood. This is pretty powerful for smelling such a tiny flower.

In January 2014, West Virginia's Wheeling Jesuit University showed peppermint and/or cinnamon dispersed while driving increased alertness and consciousness, and it decreased fatigue and frustration. Other independent studies have shown that the scent of pine can decrease anger, and peppermint was linked to helping athletes run faster with increased performance time.

Some of the most notable contributors to the aromatherapy world in the 21st century are Marguerite Maury (1895-1968), Jean Claude Lapraz, M.D., Robert Tisserand and Gabriel Mojay. In the 1950's Marguerite Maury, a biochemist, linked aromatherapy with the beauty and cosmetic industry.

She won many international awards for integrating aromatherapy into the cosmetic world, and established several aromatherapy clinics in Europe *(http://www.skininc.com/skinscience/ingredients/The-Science-of-Essential-Oils-303299761.html# sthash.M45PDpS1.dpuf)*.

Jean Claude Lapraz, M.D., a French Medical Doctor, is a world-renowned pioneer in the field of clinical phytotherapy and aromatherapy, and the co-innovator of Endobiogeny. He studied the work of Dr. Valnet and further developed his work in the 1970's. Endobiogeny is an innovative medical concept based on a refined view of the neuro-endocrine system that integrates classical medicine with herbs and supplements, essential oils, dietary and lifestyle modifications to create a truly holistic treatment approach to illnesses of the body and mind. His work is being further employed and developed at the Endobiogenic Integrative Medical Center in Idaho, USA.

In the mid 1970's, Robert Tisserand, an English Aromatherapist and educator, started Tisserand Aromatherapy. He has since authored numerous books including the 1977 publication of the *Art of Aromatherapy* and 2013 second edition, *Essential Oil Safety: A Guide for Health Care professionals*. He is involved in several national and international aromatherapy organizations and a leader in essential oil safety practices.

Gabriel Mojay has been in the wellness industry since the mid-late 1970's. He was involved with several international aromatherapy organizations which paved the way for the International Federation of Professional Aromatherapist (IFPA) in 2002, in which he was a founding co-chair. He authored the book *Aromatherapy for Healing the Spirit* and is deeply embedded in the awareness, advancements and community of aromatherapy.

In the mid 1990's, Dr. Jane Buckle, Ph.D., R.N., an English critical care nurse, Aromatherapist and educator, pioneered the 'M' Technique®, an alternative to massage therapy using slow stroking movements for critical care patients. She has made prominent strides in the aromatherapy industry and is a key advocate for published scientific studies.

Another significant contributor to the aromatherapy industry that has made incredible strides over the last 25 years by sharing the power of aromatherapy for mental, emotional, physical, spiritual and soul healing, is Dr. Bruce Berkowsky, N.M.D., M.H., H.M.C. He has conducted many, official and unofficial, research studies showing a strong connection to deep, soul-level emotional healing through the use of aromatherapies to help people connect to their true self. You can discover more of his work at www.NaturalHealthScience.com.

Future
The future is extremely bright for aromatherapy. It is already becoming a part of our everyday living habits in current society. Just about anyone you ask, could give you some experience they have had in their lifetime involving aromatherapy, and the memories they revisited via this powerful sense of smell. We are seeing more science published monthly at www.PubMed.com on the olfaction process, receptor functions and scent influences on physiology and psychology. These findings are demonstrating the powerful effect aromatherapy has on the body and mind, and helping to integrate it as an integrative modality in the natural health process.

But how will aromatherapy be used to impact our lives in the future? Will we see new technology and devices being created to more efficiently employ aromatherapy in a multitude of locations? A more widespread use of essential oils in medical facilities as a regular protocol? More natural and authentic perfumes that are less adulterated and more pure to the plant essence (as in ancient times)? An integration in foods and beverages as a pH alkalizer, flavor enhancer, digestive support and preservative? Science is showing us that this is already happening and gaining momentum. We will continue to see an increase in science-based discoveries exemplifying the profound therapeutic properties of many more essential oils for mind-body health concerns. A unique invention I recently stumbled upon are "smencils", scented pencils, for enhancing learning and cognitive functions *(http://www.wju.edu/about/adm_news_story.asp?iNewsID=4041 &strBack=/services/Default.asp)*. What role will you play in bringing aromatherapy into our next generation?

From body sprays and gels, perfumes, laundry detergents and room deodorizers to integrative mental health protocols, hospice care and emotional healing boosters, we will see aromatherapy become more of a household name just like Kleenex™ and Post-its™. I envision aromatherapy ventilation and shower systems will become a standard feature in residential, commercial and school architecture. There will be a standard aromatherapy option in all vehicles – cars, trucks, trains, planes and buses. There will be more free-standing aromatherapy oxygen bars as well as integrated ones in retailers, businesses and hospitals.

Safety Guidelines

Essential oils are approximately 100 times more potent than their actual herb form. Although pure essential oils are extractions from a natural substance, they can still be dangerous and harmful if proper precautions and education are not exercised. There are several factors to consider before using essential oils, such as age, health condition, sensitivities and allergies, essential oil quality, essential oil chemistry, dilution ratios and application methods. This book covers these topics and more.

JennScents, Inc. adopts the National Association of Holistic Aromatherapy (NAHA) and International Federation of Professional Aromatherapists (IFPA) safety guidelines for general, pregnancy, eye and dermal safety. These can be viewed at www.NAHA.org and www.IFPAroma.org. Let's discuss some safety guidelines to incorporate into your personal and professional aromatherapy regimen.

Essential oils interact within the body in three ways – physiological, psychological and biochemical. Physiologically, they have an effect on body functions. Psychologically, when we smell a scent, the limbic system is activated, thus triggering chemical and neurotransmitter responses that can affect, adjust, shift and inspire mood and behavior. *(Buchbauer, 1993; Johnson, 2011; Shibamoto et al, 2010).* Biochemically, when essential oils are metabolized in the bloodstream, they interact with enzymes, hormones and other processes.

General

- Keep all essential oils out of the reach of children, pets and those with cognitive impairments and deficiencies.
- Essential oils are not water-soluble, they are fat-soluble. This means that the essential oils will not mix or disperse in water but will mix with carrier oils (olive, grapeseed, etc.).
- Most essential oils require a carrier and should not be used directly on the skin. For those essential oils that are being used neat, test patch on the skin before use on a large area.
- Keep a carrier close by when blending or using essential oils on the skin. If there is an irritation, you want to dilute it in a fat soluble base such as olive oil, grapeseed oil or milk.
- If you are working with someone who has high blood pressure, avoid

"heating" or "stimulating" essential oils such as thyme, rosemary and oregano as they may increase blood pressure. Ylang ylang is a good choice for those with hypertension.

- If you have or you are working with someone who has a serious health condition such as heart disease, have them consult their physician before using any essential oils.

- Use caution with essential oil exposure during pregnancy, especially in the first trimester and high-risk pregnancies. According to the International Federation of Professional Aromatherapists *(www.IFPAroma.org)*, certain essential oils are contraindicated due to the nature of their chemical components, which may be too strong (and unnecessary) for a pregnant client, bearing in mind that the skin and placental barrier are more delicate and sense of smell more heightened. More safety guidelines and information can be found on the Safety Page at www.NAHA.org. The few essential oils I feel comfortable using are lavender, chamomile, frankincense, patchouli, citrus oils and peppermint for nausea in a very small amount.

- Citrus essential oils are photosensitive (phototoxic). This means that they may cause pigmentation and discoloration to the skin when exposed to direct sunlight within three to four hours after topical application. Therefore, avoid direct sunlight and tanning beds after topical use of these oils.

- Internal use is a very important topic. One should only considered this application when working with a highly trained, professional Aromatherapist. Much education and training should be employed as large amounts can be intoxicating, harmful and disturb internal membranes. Some essential oils should never be ingested due to their toxicity on organs, especially with certain medical conditions.

- Essential oils are highly flammable substances and should be kept away from direct contact with flames, such as candles, fire, matches, cigarettes, and gas cookers.

- Only use 100% pure essential oils from a reputable and experienced company.

Contraindications & Toxicity

These contraindications should be considered with everyone experiencing some type of health concern. These precautions are not to alarm you, but rather educate you on proper and responsible use and employment of aromatherapy.

- Those with serious health conditions such as cardiovascular and neurological issues, should consult their physician and pharmacist before beginning any essential oil therapy for possible interactions.
- Avoid sunlight exposure after topical use of citrus essential oils to avoid skin irritations and pigmentation.
- Those taking blood thinner medications should use caution with essential oils such as cinnamon, sage and hyssop. Thyme essential oil may slow down blood clotting.
- Asthma may be induced by certain essential oils such as thyme. Also, do not use steam inhalation as the heat and steam may aggravate the mucosal membranes.
- Some oils should be avoided with Epilepsy such fennel, sage, rosemary, camphor and hyssop.
- As a precaution, those with estrogenic cancers may want to avoid certain essential oils with estrogenic mimicking properties such as geranium, rose and clary sage.
- Those taking statin medications should avoid essential oils that could cause hepatotoxicity, especially ingestion, such as pennyroyal, thuja, anise, clove and wintergreen.
- Those with liver disease, should use caution with essential oils that are hepatotoxic such as anise, basil, bay laurel, cinnamon, clove, fennel, nutmeg, oregano, tarragon and thyme.
- Pine is contraindicated with significant prostate concerns.
- Those taking acne medications should avoid topical use of citrus oils on their skin.
- Nephrotoxic oils should be avoided with those experiencing kidney and renal failure, such as bay laurel, cinnamon, clove, coriander, juniper, sandalwood and pine. Small quantities should only be diffused for a short period of time.
- For those with glaucoma, caution should be used as some essential oils may raise intraocular pressure such as cypress, hyssop, tarragon and thyme.

Quality Assurance

How can you tell the difference between a pure, unadulterated essential oil and a synthetic one? Well, your nose usually knows. Pure essential oils can produce therapeutic effects or responses in addition to a nice, pleasant smell. The molecular structure of a 100% pure, unadulterated or diluted essential oil is small and mirrors that of the body. Therefore, your body recognizes it, accepts it, can use it and knows how to dispose of it. Synthetic fragrances or adulterated essential oils on the other hand, have a much larger molecular structure that cannot penetrate a cell, lining or the skin in most cases. These tend to confuse the body, serving as a toxin or congesting since the body does not know how to use it or dispose of it. Your mood may feel better with some synthetic fragrances, but they don't have therapeutic value such as increasing the oxygen uptake at the cellular level, hence compromising the lymphatic system's ability to function optimally. Overall, pure essential oils can penetrate the wall of dying cells to stimulate immune responses, something I've coined as "CPR for the cells".

In the wars of "sales" and "discounts", 100% pure, unadulterated essential oils tend to cost more upfront. When you look at the overall picture, they will actually cost less in the long run, as your immune system will be stronger and capable of functioning at its optimal level. You will also need less of a pure essential oil as the effects will have a positive impact to the body and mind. In addition, most people have allergies and sensitivities to synthetic fragrances. 100% pure, unadulterated essential oils do not have a protein structure, so many people (not everyone) do not have allergy response to the real thing.

Testing

Pure essential oils have chemical constituents that produce various therapeutic effects. There are testing devices, such as the Gas Chromatography, that can separate the various therapeutic constituents of a given essential oil. This is the most common and accurate test, and produces a "fingerprint" of the essential oil to ensure it contains the constituents desired for the highest quality oil.

Harvesting & Production

Proper harvesting is essential to the quality of a pure essential oil. Certain factors play a role in the therapeutic properties an essential oil possesses. The plant, flower, bush or tree must be grown in the proper pH soil, during specific climate conditions and in the best location in the world that produces and cultivates the highest chemical constituents within that plant. The plant material must be harvested at the appropriate time of day, month and year using the proper extraction method. These measures can dictate different chemical molecular structures within an essential oil. For example, lavender essential oil from the seed matures slowly but produces a rich, more complete essential oil versus lavender grown and cultivated from clippings. Most essential oils today are cultivated rather than grown wild, due to its control to meet production supply and demand. We'll soon discuss chemotypes, the designation for these locational plants that produce different essential oils with different chemical composition.

In Europe and Asia, they have the highest essential oil production at date. China, for example, is popular for their eucalyptus and jojoba production because of their good climate conditions particular to these plants. Some species are endangered as they have been over-harvested, such as sandalwood and rosewood. The government has restrictions now on rosewood that require a new tree be planted for each one harvested. It takes about 30-50 years to get the inner bark and heartwood to distill as the trees are typically 20-25 years old before oil is present. Lavender used to be harvested by hand but due to high demands today, much of it is harvested by a tractor. This essential oil is the most adulterated oil on the market. Another interesting fact, myrrh essential oil takes the longest to distill.

Plant Identification, Botany & Chemotypes
Understanding the botany and signature traits of a plant can give insight to its structure, purpose, benefits and relationship with the others oils and the environment. Knowing the plant in which an essential oil is derived can help you assess its therapeutic properties and more effectively formulate and create an aromatherapy blend to meet specific needs. It is helpful to be able to distinct one plant from another, such as its name, geography and appearance. Plant Classification, also known as taxonomy, helps avoid confusion when researching or purchasing essential oils. Latin and common names of essential oils, help avoid confusion in their therapeutic properties. You'll want to consider the family, genus, species, subspecies, hybrids, cultivars and variety (respectively), as different plants yield different therapeutic qualities. Latin names are based on a classification system developed in the 1700's. The names are always italicized, the first word is capitalized and the remainder of the names are lower case. They will tell you a plant's origin, and chemotype, meaning different variations of a plant that produce different qualities and properties. The chemotypes can further enlighten you on an oil's performance and properties. Lavender for instance, grown in France will differ from lavender grown in Florida. Some examples of

chemotypes are:

- Lavender: *Lavandula angustifolia or officinalis, Lavandula latifolia, Lavandula fragrans* (aka lavendin)
- Juniper: *Juniperus virginiana, Juniperus communis, Juniperus sabina*
- Chamomile: *Anthemis nobilis, Chamaemelum nobile, Matricaria chamomilla or retutita, Ormensis mixta or Anthemis mixta*
- Rosemary: *Rosemarinus officinalis, Rosemarinus officinalis verbenone (safest rosemary species for high blood pressure)*

Choosing Reputable Supplies and Sources

When using aromatherapy, it is important to have high-quality, credible and pure essential oils and carriers. Only the purest of oils will deliver the therapeutic properties and benefits you are seeking. Does the supplier obtain their essential oil and plant materials from a reputable and sustainable farm, with proper testing, pesticide and chemical-free and follow strict harvesting practices? A company's standards can tell you a lot about their ethics and purpose.

What is Aromatherapy?

To me, aromatherapy is an art and a science, working together to bring harmony within. Aromatherapy has been defined as the use of 100% pure essential oils to influence, affect, modify, change, shift and alter mood, emotions, physical functions, behaviors, actions, responses and our environment. Effects can be provoked in less than a second, guiding our body and mind to react.

It is a powerful tool that is complementary to numerous healing alternatives such as herbal supplements, massage, facials, chiropractic care, acupuncture, reflexology, reiki, other natural health trades and even traditional medicine. More importantly, aromatherapy can help the human body and pets heal itself by supplying the body's cells with energy, strengthen the immune system and activate a positive attitude. Our bodies have amazing, resilient abilities and using 100% pure essential oils can provide the fuel necessary for a healthy, optimal and higher quality of well-being - physically, emotionally, mentally and spiritually.

In emotional healing, it can help one connect with deep-seated, past events to recognize them, accept them and work through them to achieve emotional freedom. It helps one own the emotions rather than the emotions owning them. This will make it easier to release the emotions.

What are Essential Oils?

Essential oils are the "liquid" form and life essence of herbal plant matter. They are derived from the bark, flowers, fruits, leaves, roots, resins, seeds, stems and twigs. Although there are over 500,000 different plants available, only about 3-4% of them can produce a pure, genuine and authentic essential oil (*http://www.ncbi.nlm.nih.gov/pmc/articles/PMC88925/*). These essential oils are made up of chemical components that determine their therapeutic effects. These can be viewed in a gas chromatography test, which reveals the chemical constituents present to ensure it is indeed an unadulterated essential oil.

Essential oils possess numerous healing properties such as antibacterial, antiviral, antifungal and antiseptic. They can assist various body systems to function optimally and efficiently. For example, red mandarin offers nourishment and support to the adrenals and nervous system function, tea tree offers antifungal support and roman chamomile offers antispasmodic relief for intestinal cramping and muscle spasms. Furthermore, pure essential oils can destroy foreign invaders without killing probiotics.

Folklore

Knowing detailed historical facts, traditions, tales, beliefs and myths can enlighten you and strengthen your aromatherapy skills when choosing essential oils to integrate and create blends that match your specific goals, purpose and needs. It is through this understanding of a plant's ancestry, upbringing, personality, behavior, character and appearance that you can tell a great deal about its performance as it relates to human and pet therapy. When exploring a plant's portrait, some characteristics to contemplate are the shape and color of the flower, leaf or roots, soil composition, growth span and weather conditions for optimal growing and harvesting.

With soil composition and weather conditions, for example, some plants thrive best in dry, hot, sandy soil, whereas others may flourish best with wet, cool and damp soil. When evaluating this, you can apply this "signature" to the client you are creating an aromatherapy blend for...you, your family, friends, clients or pets. If someone is better when they are exposed to heat, then you may want to consider using cinnamon and/or rosemary. For someone better for cool temperatures, consider peppermint and/or juniper. For those with alternating better for warmth and better for cold, blue chamomile would be a good essential oil choice.

Extraction Methods

Extraction of essential oils dates back to the ancient history of the Egyptians, Persians, Chinese and Indian cultures. Over the years, specialty equipment and expertise that produces higher yields have been created and perfected. Let's take a closer look at six different extraction method for essential oils.

The first is steam distillation. It is the most widely recognized and employed process due to its efficiency, high quality and therapeutic results. Almost all of your essential oils should be steam distilled except for your citrus oils, which are produced via the expression process and those hard to yield oils. Water Distillation is another form used for oils that are heat sensitive such as neroli and rose. This is slower process and can only be used with those oils that can withstand long exposure to hot water without compromising its integrity.

Second are Hydrosols, which are pure natural water produced during the distillation process. When distilled, steam softens the plant matter, releasing a vapor. The vapor mixes with the steam and again separates only after it has cooled. This separation gives two layers – essential oil and hydrosol (hydrolat) or floral water (from flowers). These cannot be synthetically manufactured in a lab as their composition is different from essential oils. You can use hydrosols diluted or undiluted and they are generally safe for internally use when properly educated. They are great to use in skin care, with high-risk health concerns, prescription use and daily hygiene routines. Their properties will vary depending on the plant distilled. If you want more education on hydrosols I recommend a great book by Ann Harmon called *Harvest to Hydrosol* (2015).

The third extraction process is called cold expression. Only citrus oils are derived with this process via sensitive machines used to extract the essential oils from the rind or peel, not the pulp. Often, the fruit material is soaked in cool to warm water to soften it or a sponge is used to collect the oil before placing in the chamber.

Fourth is Solvent Extraction, a gentle process used with those oils that have low volatility and yield low concentrations of oil. Liquid solvents are used to get an extract, which is then distilled with gentle heat to boil off the solvent. A disadvantage with this process is that some of the waxes and plant pigments are extracted along with the plant matter into the solution. When extracted from a solid or semi-solid resin, such as a cut into tree bark, it is called a resinoid. These are often used as fixatives. If there is no resin, but rather plant material such as leaves, flowers and roots, it is called a concrete, leaving it a wax-like solid. These are harder to blend with and must either be warmed or combined with a carrier oil such as fractionated coconut oil, to blend with. Absolutes are made from concretes, which are warmed with some alcohol, heated just enough to melt it and then stirred. The essential oil will then separate from the concrete (wax). This solution is then chilled, filtered and the alcohol is removed by distillation in a vacuum at a low temperature to produce the absolute. This is considered to be the highest concentration achieved from a natural fragrance that can possibly be obtained. According to David Stewart, in his book *The Chemistry of Essential Oils Made Simple*, absolutes should not be classified as essential oils, but rather its own classification of "absolute" or "essence". Further, these type of oils should not be ingested due to the solvent residue which may be present from the process.

The fifth is the Carbon Dioxide method which is a fairly new process. It requires a stainless steel, closed chamber with a lower temperature than distillation, decreasing the affect heat has on the oil. It is a fairly quick process however uses expensive equipment. Only small amounts of an oil can be produced at a time with this method.

The final extraction process is called enfleurage. This process was one of the first used to create aromatic fragrances in ancient history. Flowers were placed in odorless and purified solid fats or oils that absorbed the essential oils such as monoi oil. This method takes a long time.

Chemistry
Essential oils typically contain about 100 different types of volatile molecules. An essential oil performs in a holistic manner and not just one constituent dictates the action of that oil, it is the combination of those constituents that create the therapeutic power. The chemistry of essential oils are broken down into main groups based on the predominating chemical components and structure. These groups of molecules can determine predictable properties. Many essential oils may fit into several chemical families, however I'd look at the top two to three families for the most potency and power.

One thing I have noticed is that chemistry is not unanimous across the board. Different varieties and different regions produce a different chemical make-up. That's why one supplier's description may vary from another. Harvesting and manufacturing plays a huge role, as well as the age and parts of the plant used. After reviewing much chemistry from an assortment of sources, I found some similarities and commonalities, but also varying information. So, in my chemistry section for each essential oil profile, I have listed the most common components found, understanding that this may vary a bit depending on your source. These listed are prevalent in my current sources and referenced from *The Chemistry of Essential Oils Made Simple* (2006) by David Stewart (most comprehensive), *Essential Chemistry for Safe Aromatherapy* (2002) by Sue Clark and www.Pubmed.com.

Using chemistry to create blends can be fun for some, and intimidating for others. As a good Aromatherapist, you should at least be familiar with essential oil chemistry and its role in the blend. It can lend an extra layer of therapeutic results, and guide you on formulating safely. Looking at the last few letters of a chemical constituents name can give you a clue as to which family it belongs, then you can match that families characteristics with your blends purpose.

Chemical Constituent Name Recognition			
Terpenes	'ene'	Esters	'-lyl acetate'
Alcohols	'ol'	Ethers	'ol, ole'
Phenols	'ol'	Lactones	'lactone'
Aldehydes	'aldehyde'	Oxides	'oxide'
Ketones	'one'	Carboxyl Acids	'acids'

Almost all molecules found in essential oils are carbon, hydrogen and oxygen. The chemistry of an essential oil is determined by two factors - the extraction process and its genetic molecular structure. There are two principle categories of chemical constituents present in essential oils - unsaturated hydrocarbons (terpenes) and oxygenated compounds. Few essential oils do contain saturated hydrocarbons, such as *Rosa damascena*.

Saturated Hydrocarbons (Alkanes)
The simplest family of the hydrocarbons, alkanes contain only a single joining bond. They are called saturated hydrocarbons because there is a hydrogen in every possible location *(http://hyperphysics.phy-astr.gsu.edu/hbase/organic/alkane.html)*. Examples are methane, ethane, propane and butane.

Alkenes and Alkynes are both unsaturated hydrocarbons. Unsaturated hydrocarbons are hydrocarbons that have double or triple covalent bonds (sharing of electron pairs between atoms) between adjacent carbon atoms. Alkenes have one or more double bonds. Alkynes have one or more triple bonds *(Tisserand, 2002)*.

Unsaturated Hydrocarbons (Terpenes)
Most chemical constituents found in essential oils are terpenoids. These consists of hydrogens and carbons. Steam distillation extracts are the only volatile and water insoluble constituents such as terpenes and terpenoid compounds (hydrocarbons). When essential oils are extracted with solvents, the absolutes contain very little to no terpenes. Terpenoids have carbons in multiples of five. For example, 5 carbon atoms are called hemiterpenes; 10 carbon atoms are called monoterpenes; 15 carbon atoms are called sesquiterpenes; 20 carbon atoms are called diterpenes; 30 carbon atoms are called triterpenes; and 40

carbon atoms are called tetraterpenes. The number depends on the pH of the distillation process. Terpenes (especially monoterpenes) are found in almost every essential oil and end in "ene".

Monoterpene examples are citrus oils (limonene), palo santo, pine needle (α-pinene/β-pinene), angelica (phellandrene, sabinene) and juniper (α-terpinene/γ-terpinene). These are generally top and upper middle notes. They are mild but can have some occasional skin irritation or dryness, so a carrier is recommended. They are known to stimulate toxin removal from the body and reduce tissue irritation. They have a high volatility, evaporate and oxidize quickly when exposed to air, heat and light. They possess properties of antiseptic, tonic, stimulating, decongestant and antiviral.

Sesquiterpenes are 15 carbon atoms, and like monoterpenes, they too are found in many essential oils. These are the largest group of terpenes and often found in roots and woods. These are generally middle to base notes, and are potent, so small amounts can produce a profound influence and strong odor. Examples are atlas cedar, German chamomile (bisabolene/chamazulene), rose and many flower oils (farnesene), sandalwood and clove (caryophyllene). Sesquiterpenes are generally antiseptic, anti-inflammatory, antispasmodic, calming, slightly hypotensive and sedative (i.e.caryophyllene).

Diterpenes are 20 carbon atoms. They are generally antifungal and antiviral. They may have a balancing effect on the endocrine system. Examples are white camphor, clary sage, jasmine and tea tree.

Oxygenated Compounds
Oxygenated compounds consists of hydrogen, carbon and oxygen. They include alcohol, esters, aldehydes, ketones, lactones and ethers. This functional group determines a property's strength. Oxygen, infuses "life" into the essential oils.

Alcohols
Alcohols, not rubbing alcohol, are most beneficial and have a pleasant fragrance. They offer germicide, antiseptic, energizing and deodorant properties. Lavender (linalool), palmarosa, eucalyptus (terpineol) and rosewood are examples. There are three subcategories within the Alcohol family – Monoterpenols, Sesquiterpenols and Diterpenols. You will commonly find components such as linalool in the Labiatae (mint), Lauraceae (laurel) and Rutaceae (citrus) families.

Monoterpene alcohols are non-irritating, have low toxicity and irritation thus great for children, elderly and those with sensitivities. They are antiseptic, antifungal, antiviral, antibacterial and energizing. They are typically cooling oils. Examples are citronella and rose (geraniol), peppermint (menthol) and palmarosa.

Sesquiterpene alcohols are not common in most essential oils. They are found in many base notes and offer anti-allergenic, hepatic and anti-inflammatory properties. Examples are rose (farnesol), sandalwood (α-santalol), German chamomile (α-bisabolol) and patchouli. Diterpenols are known to have a balancing effect on the endocrine system such as clary sage (sclareol).

Phenols
Phenols are best to use in low concentrations for a short period of time, as excessive amounts may irritate the liver, mucosal membranes and skin. They are antiseptic, antibacterial, antioxidant, anti-infectious and stimulating to the nervous and immune systems. Examples are clove, wintergreen, certain chemotypes of thyme (thymol) and oregano (carvacrol). Phenols are high in eugenol, which have blood thinning properties, thus proper caution should be taken.

Aldehydes
Aldehydes are often viewed as a stronger alcohol but milder ketone, and typically ends in "al". They produce a citrus-like fragrance, often lemon-like. They are unstable, oxidize quickly and can cause skin irritation if not diluted in a carrier. They offer antifungal, antiseptic, antibacterial, calming, anti-inflammatory and sedative properties, so a good choice for stress relief. Examples are eucalyptus citriodora (citronellal), cassia, lemongrass (citral) and melissa. An interesting note, lemon has a greater concentration of terpenes versus aldehydes.

Ketones
Ketones are not predominantly used as essential oils. They have a specifically strong aroma and offer analgesic, mucolytic (dissolve mucus and fats), expectorant, cell and tissue regeneration, anti-inflammatory, and vulnerary properties. They typically end in "one". Examples are rosemary (verbenone), spearmint, camphor and pennyroyal (pulegone). Excessive use can be neurotoxic (most toxic are hyssop [pinocamphone], thuja and wormwood [thujone]), so it is contraindicated with epilepsy. Use sparingly with small children.

Esters
Esters are most wide spread, balancing and safest to use of all the chemical families. It has a pleasant, fruity smell. They are balancing to nervous system,

and offer soothing, antispasmodic, antiseptic, analgesic, anti-inflammatory and sedative properties. They typically end in "yl" or "ate". Examples are Roman chamomile, lavender, helichrysum, petitgrain and wintergreen. Chamomile actually contains a number of esters not commonly found in other oils. A couple to use caution with are birch and wintergreen (neurotoxic in high amounts).

There is a subcategory called Carboxylic Acids, which reacts with alcohol to form esters. A few essential oils contain this group in their chemistry, such as salicylic acid, cinnamic acid and benzoic acid.

Ethers
Most ethers in essential oils are phenolic ethers. They are not common but have distinctive licorice smell. They offer antispasmodic, digestive, soothing and carminative properties. The only important ones are anise (anethol), clove (eugenol), basil, fennel and tarragon (methyl carvacrol).

Lactones
More recently, we are finding more oils in the lactone class. Lactones often end in "in" but can also end in "one". Lactones are a strong mucolytic, such as inula and catnip, however excessive amounts may cause neurotoxicity and skin irritation. They may also be blood thinning in high amounts so use caution. They also offer expectorant, hypotensive and uplifting yet sedating benefits. Coumarins are a type of lactone, and include Bergaterpene (furocoumarin free).

Oxides
Oxides are derived from alcohols. They keep the alcohol name and add "oxide", or 1,8-cineole (eucalyptol). They possess expectorant, mucolytic, antiviral, decongestant and digestive stimulating properties. They have a stable, camphor-like scent such as eucalyptus, rosemary and tea tree. Chemical components include bisabolol oxide, cineole, pinene oxide, linalool oxide.

Aromatherapy Physiology: Mental, Emotional, Physical & Soul Health

Our sense of smell perpetuates an affect faster than any of our other senses. This is because the nose, commonly referred to as the "external brain", has a direct pathway to the brain. It does not have to be processed by the spinal cord or digestive tract to elicit a response, like all of our other senses. Thus, the effect on our mental, physical and emotional physiology is instantaneous and takes less than the snap of a finger.

Aromatherapy allows us to connect, channel, shift and heal emotions within ourselves on all levels, simultaneously. When we smell particular scents, it can bring peace and comfort or provide energy and vitality. Scents are made up of constituents, or characteristics (like DNA) that make them unique. Their "appearance" is represented in properties, just as a person would have blonde, black or red hair. Just like people, they have their own personality and will inspire specific feelings and thoughts when smelled. They work great individually but also are wonderful when combined with other essential oils. You can target a specific issue by reviewing the traits each essential oil possesses and then assembling your "team" to conquer that goal, just like in sports. Sports teams seek the best "players" to accomplish a sports goal. You will do the same thing in aromatherapy, choose the best essential oils to make up your aromatherapy blend to accomplish your health goal.

Aromatherapy is truly a universal resource for everyone, and everything, engaging the mind to strength concentration and focus, enhance response time and cognitive abilities. It can alert us by smelling bad food before we eat it and to engage our fight or flight system if we smell smoke coming from a fire. On an emotional level, scents trigger the olfaction process to acknowledge a scent, accept it, differentiate it and allow it to provoke a response. On a physical level, essential oils are absorbed into mucosal linings, the bloodstream and the lymph (in less than three seconds) to respond to physical concerns and disharmonies. The Gut helps the body further deliver the scent's purpose to the appropriate organs, muscles, membranes and systems. This is why the Gut-Brain connection is so important, to assess and take action. Your gut and brain are actually created out of the same type of tissue but are separated in the fetal development. The brain turns into central nervous system and the gut into the enteric nervous system, located in the gastrointestinal tract. They are connected by the vagus nerve, the tenth cranial nerve that runs from your brain stem down to your abdomen, connecting your two brains – head to gut. More and more science is being conducted and published every day showing how we are truly mind-heart-gut beings and that all must communicate in unison for optimal health *(http://www.scientificamerican.com/article/gut-second-brain/)*.

Our bodies must interconnect and intercommunicate continuously for messages to be accurately delivered to the proper places to initiate organ function and for nutrients to be absorbed, assimilated, utilized and excreted optimally. Aromatherapy facilitates these connections for overall whole body healthy functions. Our head (thought assessment center) must be in alignment and connect with the heart (feeling center) and gut (action center) for optimum performance. They should all work in agreement, and rely on one another. When there is a break down in this communication system, health imbalances start to occur and manifest with ongoing disharmony.

Mental: Head, Brain & Mind (Thought Assessment Center)
Our head houses the brain, mind and thoughts, and is structured to protect them from harm and trauma. This allows the brain function to activate the mind to assess a situation and react accordingly. Once thoughts have been assessed, they are then communicated to the gut, via the heart for action to transpire.

Our brain is amazing! It is only about 2% of our total body but contains approximately 98% of the body's nerve cells or neurons, which specialize in carrying messages throughout the body. Essential oils can help this messenger process deliver information more accurately, effectively and efficiently. It is also comprised of 70% water and 50% (good) fat by dry weight. This is important to know so we can hydrate our brain with water, minerals and good fats for it to operate successfully. Having a vehicle such as aromatherapy to assist in driving these nutrients deep within the brain is very beneficial to enhance hydration levels, offer cellular and brain function support as well as neurotransmission delivery. As I previously stated, essential oils are like "CPR" for the cells and can resuscitate oxidized and oxidizing cells. They are also fat soluble, so diluting them in a fat soluble carrier is key to helping them serve the brain.

Whereas the brain is the physical anatomy that permits cognitive processes, the mind is defined as the set of cognitive faculties that occur, enabling consciousness, perception, thinking, judgement and memory. It's where wisdom is balanced with understanding, conflict balanced with contradiction, and the ability to recognize right from wrong. When the mind is overburdened, we experience absent-mindedness, confusion, disorientation and mental fatigue.

The brain communicates via the autonomic and central nervous systems and the limbic systems. An imbalance of the mind with miscommunication to the body may cause an inability to cope and manage emotions, actions and reactions for any given situation. It may shift our responses into a reactive mode that forces us to make quick, uneducated and haste decisions that may lead to disarray, confusion and disharmony. The nervous system may eventually become exhausted and depleted of sufficient nutrients and vitamins, especially B vitamins which are necessary for stress management and head-heart-gut communication. Most impairments in our physical, mental and emotional systems have been scientifically linked to inflammation, and more specifically, in the intestines *(http://www.ncbi.nlm.nih.gov/pubmed/16320856)*. Furthermore, this has been shown to contribute to mental deficiencies such as neurotransmitter malfunction and depression *(http://www.ncbi.nlm.nih.gov/pubmed/21893478)*.

The Olfaction Process & Limbic System
Olfaction simply means the sense of smell. It takes a faster, unfiltered route than any of our other senses. It allows us to take in a scent as it travels through the nose, detect it and dissolve it in our mucosal membrane, pass it to the olfactory nerves, called cilia, then to the olfactory bulb where it then relays information to the limbic system and triggers a response. Let's look at the life of a scent molecule in more detail.

1. A scent enters into the nose.
2. It then travels along the cilia, which are hair-like structures at the tips of olfactory nerves.
3. Next it will penetrate and dissolve the aroma vapor in the mucus membranes of the olfactory epithelium located at the roof of the nasal cavity. Then sending it to specialized receptor cells called olfactory receptor neurons that will detect the odor and relay information.
4. These olfactory receptors transmit the scent information to the olfactory bulb, located at the back of the nose. These receptors can perceive thousands of different odors. The chemistry of certain scent molecules will trigger certain receptors to respond in a certain way, hence relaxation, invigoration, antiviral, etc.
5. The Olfactory bulb is the scent recognition and processing center with sensory receptors attached to the brain. It sits on the bottom of the brain,

just above the nasal cavity and sends messages directly to the limbic system and conscious thought.

6. From here, a response is generated via the limbic system, telling you how to respond to stimuli, whether it be emotions, memories, thoughts or behaviors. We'll discuss how the heart and gut gets involved in just a few minute.

Just think, our sense of taste is limited to sweet, sour, bitter, pungent, astringent and salty. But our sense of smell has been reported to have over 10,000 different odors it can detect *(Richard Axel, 1995)*. A more recent study from March 2014 states that "humans can discriminate at least 1 trillion olfactory stimuli (scents)" *(http://www.ncbi.nlm.nih.gov/pubmed/24653035)*, far greater than any of our other senses. Smells can stimulate memories of past events, connecting us to remember what we were doing, what we were wearing and what we were thinking at a specific moment in time. Olfaction is the one place where the nervous system is in constant, direct contact with the external environment.

The Limbic System, known as the "oldest" part of brain, is comprised of a set of structures above the brain stem and under the cerebrum, in the middle of the brain. It helps the limbic and cerebral cortex's communicate and relay messages. It is the system where thinking and analytical development occurs and is responsible for our olfaction ability, emotions, behavior, motivation, arousal, learning and memory. It is made up of the following:

Olfactory bulb: Processes and transmits scent information from the nose to the brain. Excessive toxic inhalation exposure, traumatic brain injury and other damage to this area can result in anosmia, the loss of sense of smell.

Olfactory cortex: Receives sensory information from the olfactory bulb for odor identification. According to Candace B. Pert, Ph.D. in the *Molecules of Emotion*, "the efficiency of the filtering process, which chooses what stimuli we pay attention to at any given moment, is determined by the quantity and quality of the receptors at the nodal points (regions of high concentrations of neuropeptide receptors where information enters the nervous system)."

Hypothalamus: Attaches and sits above pituitary (aka "master gland"), just below the thalamus. It receives sensory information, regulates body temperature, emotions, hunger, sleep and sexual desire, and releases certain hormones and sends instructions to the rest of the body via the autonomic and central nervous systems.

Thalamus: Located in the center of the brain, by the cerebral cortex. Involved in sensory perception and regulation of motor functions such as movement and thinking as well as relays sensory signals (smell, sight, etc.) and information to and from the spinal cord and the cerebral cortex via hypothalamus. Interesting note, the cerebral cortex, the surface of the brain, makes up about 80% of our brain.

Hippocampus: Located under the cerebral cortex. Converts short-term memories into long-termed memories, stores them and is involved with spatial memory and learning. Damage to this area can lead to amnesia and dementia. The **Fornix** connects the hippocampus to the hypothalamus. It plays a part in memory recall and recognition.

Amygdala: Located deep within the cerebral cortex next to the hippocampus. Determines what memories are stored where, hormonal secretions, decision making and emotional responses such as fear, aggression and survival instincts (fight or flight). A study in April 2011 showed that the amygdala is related to the control of associative fear memory formation *(http://www.ncbi.nlm.nih.gov/pubmed/21471365)*.

Basal Ganglia: Located near the thalamus and hypothalamus, it receives input from the cerebral cortex and sends it to the brain stem. It is responsible for repetitive behaviors, conditioning, addictions, focus attention and movement.

References: *http://brainmind.com/OlfactoryLimbicSystem.html,* *http://www.healing-arts.org/n-r-limbic.htm, http://www.ncbi.nlm.nih.gov/pmc/articles/PMC2917081/)*

The purpose of the Limbic System is to regulate dozens of body functions such as hunger, thirst, weight, temperature, blood sugar, growth, sleeping, walking, sexual arousal, emotions, and to transform thought into action. When an essential oil contacts the limbic system, a response is generated in less than one second via inhalation and less than one to three seconds via skin application. Your body is smart and resilient and will take in the essential oils it needs to balance emotions, thoughts and mental abilities. It is important to like the smell when first addressing emotional and mental concerns so you can start to build a trusting relationship. As you work deeper on an emotional, soul and spiritual level, you may incorporate scents that may not be your favorite, but are necessary for your healing journey.

Research shows that when olfaction is intact, twice as many memories were recalled when associated with scent. Studies have shown that olfaction abilities such as odor detection and identification decrease with the aging process. Several factors have been claimed to be the culprit of this decline such as overexposure to chemicals and toxins, chronic respiratory infections, allergies, brain injuries, smoking, certain prescription medications and natural aging processes *(http://www.ncbi.nlm.nih.gov/pmc/articles/PMC2682444/)*. A June 2015 study states that "the incidence of olfactory impairment increases sharply in the eighth and ninth decades of life but the etiology of age-related olfactory decline is not well understood. Inflammation and atherosclerosis are associated with many age-related conditions and atherosclerosis has been associated with olfactory decline in middle-aged adults" *(http://www.ncbi.nlm.nih.gov/pubmed/260821788)*. Further, many diseases such as cancer and Alzheimer's have been linked to olfactory deficits and dysfunctions *(http://www.ncbi.nlm.nih.gov/pubmed/20709038)*. People with anosmia, the loss of smelling ability, report more social isolation and anhedonia (inability to feel pleasure) which can severely affect quality of life *(http://www.ncbi.nlm.nih.gov/pubmed/23875929)*. Nutritionally, further science has been done to show higher consumption of good fats such as nuts and fish may reduce the odds of olfactory impairment *(http://www.ncbi.nlm.nih.gov/pubmed/26079067)*, as it has been related to enhance circulatory and lymphatic functions.

Anosmia can be enhanced with proper nutrition, minerals, efficient elimination of waste and daily exposure to scents. Nutritionally, it has been scientifically linked to a deficiency of zinc *(http://articles.mercola.com/sites/articles/archive/2014/10/15/anosmia-loss-sense-smell.aspx)*, an important trace mineral for immunity, absorption, growth and development. Minerals in general are important for urinary and circulatory systems to function optimally. They keep things moving optimally within the body and mind, helping to eliminate wastes effectively, especially heavy metals, which can overburden the kidneys and prostate when they cannot be flushed. I have also found a connection between deficient thyroid function, so it may be worth considering.

To retrain your nose to smell again, sniff a couple of essential oils, six to ten times per nostril, once or twice a day. Rotate scents a couple times a week. I especially find the culinary scents like cinnamon, lemon, thyme and ginger most beneficial. For some people, they can start smelling again within a couple months, for other with more severe trauma to their olfactory system, it may take much longer.

Scent Science

The Proust Phenomenon is described as the sudden occurrence of a powerful memory *(http://psychologydictionary.org/proust-phenomenon/)*. This phenomenon was named after Marcel Proust, a French writer who authored a seven-volume novel about memory and time called *In Search of Lost Time*. He compiled his novels from 1909-22, first published between 1913 to 1927, and later translated into English by C. K. Scott Moncrieff in 2003. This novel discusses the themes of involuntary memories and perceptions of time. This insight gives rise to further science and comprehension of scent memories, or the place where "involuntary memories meets voluntary memories". It is elaborated in the voluntary functions of the olfactory cortex, amygdala and other scent-evoking organs.

Psychology studies have shown that memories triggered by scent can provoke a heightened intensity of emotions *(https://www.psychologytoday.com/blog/intense-emotions-and-strong-feelings/201203/emotional-memories-when-people-and-events-remain)*. "There is this unique connection between the sense of smell and the part of the brain that processes emotion," says Rachel Herz, a cognitive neuroscientist at Brown University in Providence, Rhode Island. Others studies have revealed the power of scent for memory recall. I personally like to smell a particular scent when I am studying, then smell that same scent again when I am retrieving that information to enhance my memory associations. The recall is faster and more accurate than non-scent exposure. You will be hearing much more about this in the coming years as science reveals its intricacies of our mind and body. Here is a quote that gives insight as to the depths of Marcel's novels, *In Search of Time, volumes 1-7..."I felt myself still reliving a past which was no longer anything more than the history of another person"*.

Richard Axel and Linda Buck won the 2004 Nobel Prize in Physiology or Medicine for their discoveries of odorant receptors and their relationship to the organization of the olfactory system *(1991, USA)*. They discovered a large gene family, comprised of some 1,000 different genes (3% of our genes) that give rise to an equivalent number of olfactory receptor types. These receptors are located on the olfactory receptor cells, which occupy a small area in the upper part of the nasal epithelium and detect the inhaled odorant molecules. Each olfactory receptor cell has only one type of odorant receptor, and each receptor can detect a limited number of odorant substances, therefore making them highly specialized for a few odors. The cells send thin nerve impulses directly to distinct micro domains, glomeruli, in the olfactory bulb. From these micro domains, the information is relayed further to other parts of the brain, where the information from several olfactory receptors is combined, forming a pattern. Therefore, we can consciously experience a smell and recall this olfactory memory at other times *(www.nobelprize.org/nobel_prizes/medicine/laureates/2004/press.html)*. Since then, a plethora of studies have been conducted to further their research and expound upon gene discovery and olfactory receptor functions. You can find up-to-date studies at www.PubMed.com.

Odorant Receptors and the Organization of the Olfactory System

Diagram Reference: Buck, L. and Axel, R. (1991) Cell, vol. 65, 175-187.

Mental Benefits with Aromatherapy
- Mood: citrus, floral, spicy, camphoraceous scents
    - Depression: Nervous system deficiency. Citrus (bergamot, orange), floral (jasmine, neroli, Roman chamomile) and camphor (eucalyptus, rosemary).
    - Anxiety: Nervous system excess. Citrus (bergamot), florals (rose lavender, ylang ylang), woodsy (cedar, pine) and florals (Roman chamomile, geranium).

- Nervousness: Nervous system spasms. Citrus (bergamot, orange), floral (lavender, Roman chamomile), herb (lemongrass) and camphoresque (frankincense, ravinsara).
- Panic Attacks: Spicy (cinnamon), citrus (bergamot) and floral (clary sage, melissa, ylang ylang).
- Obsessive Compulsive (uncontrolled repetitive actions and thoughts): Spicy (cinnamon, clove), citrus (grapefruit, orange), floral (clary sage, ylang ylang), woodsy and earthy (cedar, frankincense, sandalwood).
- Insomnia: Earthy and grounding (patchouli, sandalwood, vetiver) and floral (lavender, Roman chamomile).
- Cognition, learning, dementia: floral (lavender), woodsy (frankincense), spicy (cinnamon) and citrus (pink grapefruit).
  - Indecisive or Confusion: citrus (lemon), camphor (peppermint, rosemary), floral (geranium) and woodsy (cypress, patchouli).
  - Alert, accuracy, concentration: Camphor (peppermint, rosemary), citrus (lemon, orange) and floral (jasmine).
    - A Japanese study conducted by the Takasago Corporation showed that scents of lemon and jasmine reduced typing errors by 54% and 33%, respectively.
- Nightmares (usually related to parasites): Woodsy (frankincense, sandalwood) and floral (lavender, neroli).
- Addictions: Floral (clary sage, melissa), citrus (bergamot) and earthy (frankincense, vetiver).

Emotional: Heart (Feeling Center)

Emotions are e-motion, energy in motion. It requires constant movement to avoid getting stuck and being consumed by the same emotion over and over, without a break or ability to move past it. In a perfect world, we should experience an emotion, move freely with it, own it, acknowledge it, accept it, make peace with it and then let it go. It is when we don't let it go, that stuckness sets in, causing emotional imbalance that spirals into physical concerns because the mind and gut are in disharmony. Stuckness can lead to lymphatic congestion and poor circulation, both requiring movement.

We use essential oils to unlock and peel back layers, removing the clutter that burdens and surrounds us. This allows us to shed that darkness, making way for the new layers underneath to come to the forefront, to be acknowledged, addressed, forgiven and released. During your aromatherapy healing journey, new issues may arise as you peel one layer back at a time. Each layer comes with its own energy, its own issues and lessons. This gives you the opportunity to embrace it, reflect on it and use it as inspiration to carry forward. This is a continuous process to unveil each of the layers of "perception" that was built up over the years and to help tap into, and reach our inner most core, also known as the authentic self. It is only here that we all can operate at our fullest potential without the attachment of judgement and fear. I sometimes refer to this as an "aromatherapy soul cleansing". Its job is to help you release the attachment of the walls of fear. The more you cling to these negative attachments, the less you can cling to God in the truth.

Aromatherapy has an incredibly influential effect on our emotions. It can help us come to terms with and accept the emotions we are feeling, process them, understand them and help us move through them and past them. In small amounts, it can subtly shift you into a healthier state. Higher amounts, more frequently can help you dive deeper into your core, soul-level emotions, where the root of the emotional manifestations occur, but can sometimes be a little too overwhelming and overloading, so starting out with smaller amounts is what I recommend until you become comfortable with your body's emotional responses. More isn't always better in the world of aromatherapy.

It is important to note that not all scents elicit a positive response. With PTSD and negative memories, certain scents can trigger these deep, dark emotions once buried. When working though emotional issues, be mindful to discuss reactions and responses with the person you are helping...and that person might be yourself.

There is a wide spectrum of emotions that we experience throughout our lifetime such as anger, frustration, grief, guilt, fear, worry, bitterness, rejection, resentment, abandonment and so on. Different essential oils have an affinity for different emotions, and some can offer more support than others. For example, I find ravinsara to be magnificent for grief, cinnamon for abandonment and Roman chamomile for worry. However, there are some oils that have a larger spectrum of benefits, such as rose that would be good for all three grief, abandonment and worry.

Our heart is the center of our feeling domain. You may know the old saying, "the heart wants what it wants", referring to that strong, intense yearning and feeling for something that is perceived at the time to make you whole. It doesn't mean it is rational or even in alignment with your "gut instinct", but nonetheless, a powerful sensation that overrules. The majority of the time, that feeling is so strong, that we give into it, like a bad habit or addiction. Not satisfying that yearning, can take hold of our heart. This emotional pain can even present as physical pain. Often times we hear after a loss of a relation or person, someone experiences chest pains or panic attacks. This demonstrates how we are truly connected – head to heart to gut.

Emotional feelings can be triggered by genetics, hormones, neurotransmitter deficiencies, nutrient deficiencies, chemical disruptors, environmental overload and simply lack of experience in handling a situation you may never have been in before. It's not the actual stressors that produce these unhealthy responses, it's our reactions and responses to them that determine our temperament. When we go through experiences in life, sometimes those challenges are tough and demanding. It is in those moments that we learn the most about who we are, what we are capable of as well as our weaknesses. Some people view these weaknesses as failures but how can you strengthen yourself without knowing what you need to practice? Remember, it took Thomas Edison 1000 unsuccessful tries to invent one light bulb. When a reporter asked him, "How did it feel to fail 1,000 times?" Edison replied, "I didn't fail 1,000 times. The light bulb was an invention with 1,000 steps." See, it's your perception and response to the stress that can defeat you or turn yourself into your own hero. Sometimes we need support to encourage our own inspiration and motivation, which is where aromatherapy excels.

"Our greatest glory is not in never falling but in rising every time we fall." ~ Confucius

"Great success is built on failure, frustration, even catastrophe." ~ Sumner Redstone

"Failure provides the opportunity to begin again, more intelligently." ~ Henry Ford

"The fastest way to succeed is to double your failure rate." ~ Thomas Watson Sr.

"Only those who dare to fail greatly can achieve greatly." ~ Robert F. Kennedy

Emotional Benefits with Aromatherapy
- Anger, Rage, Frustration, Irritability: Camphor (peppermint), Citrus (lemon, orange), floral (lavender, Roman chamomile [my favorite], rose, ylang ylang) and woodsy (pine, cedar, helichrysum, frankincense). A December 2014 study demonstrated the relaxation benefits of inhaling orange and rose scents *(http://www.ncbi.nlm.nih.gov/pubmed/25453523)*.

- Bitterness, Resentment: Citrus (bergamot, pink grapefruit), floral (rose, palmarosa), camphor (rosemary, peppermint) and woodsy (cypress, sandalwood, patchouli).
- Emotional Distress, Exhaustion: All citrus, Spicy (cinnamon, ginger), camphor (mints, eucalyptus) and florals (lavender, geranium).
- Fear: Woodsy (frankincense, pine), floral (lavender, roman chamomile), spicy (cinnamon) and citrus (orange).
- Grief: Camphor (ravinsara, eucalyptus), floral (rose, geranium), herbal (lemongrass, marjoram).
- Guilt: Floral (clary sage, jasmine, ylang ylang) camphor (ravinsara, niaouli) and woodsy (frankincense, pine).
- Loneliness, Isolation: Citrus, floral/euphoric (clary sage, neroli), herbal (melissa, lemongrass) and sweet earthy (bay laurel, benzoin).
- Worry: Floral (Roman chamomile, lavender), woodsy (frankincense, vetiver) and all citrus.

Physical: Gut (Action Center)

As we've been discussing, the body is one being – head, heart and gut. They operate synergistically, not independently. When there is a breakdown in one system, all of the others suffer in some form whether it be emotional, mental or physical or all three. As we have been discussing, health concerns when manifested from an emotional imbalance, will exhibit a complementary physical imbalance. For example, the emotion of grief is harbored in the lungs, hence grief and respiratory ailments are related. Have you ever noticed, after a person loses a close family member, friend or pet, they seem to develop a cold, bronchitis or other respiratory discomfort? This is why whole-body, mind-body health is important.

Our gut is where the action happens. It has been scientifically shown to operate as our second brain *(http://neurosciencestuff.tumblr.com/post/38271759345/gut-instincts-the-secrets-of-your-second-brain)*. Just as the brain communicates via the central nervous system, the gut communicates via the enteric nervous system (remember, this separation of communication pathways occurs in the fetal development). It is located in the sheaths of tissue lining the esophagus, stomach, small intestine and colon. According to Dr. Keith Scott-Mumby, author of *Secrets of an Alternative Doctor*, the gut has all the neurotransmitters of the upper brain, including 90% of the body's serotonin, our happy neurotransmitter. Any inflammation in the gut causes systemic inflammation and can spread like a wild fire. Thus an anti-inflammatory diet and lifestyle can prove to be the "secret to life" *(http://unleashthethinwithin.com/leaky-gut-root-of-all-illness/)*. Many essential oils possess anti-inflammatory properties such as frankincense, chamomiles, lavender and mints. Dr. Michael Gershon, a professor of anatomy and cell biology at Columbia-Presbyterian Medical Center in New York and author of *The Second Brain*, shares that the brain in the gut plays a major role in human happiness and misery, but few people know it exists. He is conducting research studies to prove the science behind the gut brain and to debunk the "it's all in your head" phenomena. He also links the "butterflies in my stomach" sensation to anatomy and physiology *(http://www.nytimes.com/1996/01/23/science/complex-and-hidden-brain-in-gut-makes-stomachaches-and-butterflies.html)*.

When we look at the physical body, we have to give credit to the works of herbalists, Samuel Thompson and Steven Horne. Samuel Thompson, an American herbalist, who lived in the early part of the 19th century developed the Disease Tree Model. His philosophy was that until you work on the root cause or underlying causes, disease will simply manifest in another form. Steven Horne expounded upon Thompson's work to further the understanding of what the roots are and how to address them. They follow Herring's Law that you heal from the top down (head to toe), inside out (internal terrain to external appearance) and reverse order of symptoms (from present to birth).

Steven Horne, Master Herbalist and founder of the Tree of Light Institute *(www.TreeLite.com)* does a great job helping us understand our body, by comparing it to a tree. The soil is responsible for the tree and body constitution (physical and emotional makeup). It is the foundation that dictates how we will respond to our environment and is comprised of our genetic makeup. Next we have the roots which are related to our environmental stress, toxicity and nutritional deficiencies. The trunk translates to our biological terrain (internal environment) and houses our blood and lymphatic system. The branches we can view as our body system functions and require nutrients, water, oxygen, elimination and regulated temperature to survive. We typically start seeing symptoms and problems here, but the issues have been occurring for a while. Your body just reaches that point where your "cup ruteth over" and imbalances start to spill out. They usually will spill out in your weakest body system which tells us there is a breakdown in the communication lines between that system and the gut. Last, we have the twigs and leaves. These are representative of specific symptoms and health issues. You can work on the symptoms, but until you work on the root that is causing those symptoms to manifest, the problem will keep reoccurring.

Physical Benefits with Aromatherapy

- Circulation: Camphor (rosemary, black pepper), green/herbal (basil, bay laurel) and floral (ylang ylang, rose).
    - Blood pressure: rosemary stimulates blood pressure; ylang ylang calms blood pressure.
- Digestion: Gas, bloating, indigestion, reflux: Floral (Roman Chamomile), spicy (clove, nutmeg, ginger) and green/herbal (fennel, black pepper).
- Intestinal: Malabsorption, cramps, constipation, diarrhea: Floral (Roman chamomile), green/herbal (fennel, thyme), spicy (nutmeg, ginger) and camphor (peppermint).
    - Malabsorption was the root of my failing health and affects so many people. It is when you take in foods, but your body cannot physiologically absorb, assimilate and utilize the nutrients. Thus your body "starves" and cannot function optimally as it doesn't have all of the right tools to "make things run right". So failures begin to happen and we experience that by way of ailments and symptoms. A person can feel like they are hungry all of the time, not feel satisfied after eating and having trouble either gaining weight or losing weight.
- Respiratory: Congestion, cough, allergies: Camphor (eucalyptus, tea tree), woodsy (frankincense, pine), herbal (oregano, thyme) and citrus (lemon, orange).
- Structural: Bones, muscles, tendons, joints, ligament (arthritis and pain): Floral (lavender, clary sage), herbal (marjoram), camphor (eucalyptus, rosemary, peppermint) and woodsy (frankincense and cypress).
- Urinary: Swelling, edema, skin concerns (irritation, burns, bruises, insect bites, cuts, stretch marks) a urinary discomfort: herbal (helichrysum, carrot), floral (lavender, juniper) and woodsy (myrrh, patchouli, pine).

When we think about the head-heart-gut connection, or mind-body wellness, it references the communication, transportation and inter-relations between these three, simultaneously to achieve overall harmony. This relationship between the mind and body as it pertains to health was first discovered and studied in Russia more than 30 years ago. Russian scientists discovered the important role of neuro-peptides which further proved that the mind and emotions, cause a state of health and well-being, scientifically. It is the emotions that create electrical impulses that travel instantly along neural pathways, triggering the release of chemical proteins called neuro-peptides. There are more than a thousand different neuro-peptides that are the catalysts for every physiological function in the body (i.e., anger or fear triggers the release of adrenalin and cortisol). Recent scientific discoveries show that depression actually causes heart disease (*http://www.enlightenedfeelings.com/scientific_evidence.html*).

Organ Association

I first learned about organ associations from a dear friend, Dr. Kimberly Balas, Ph.D., ND. She taught about the connection between organs and corresponding emotions. She is the "queen" of biochemical blood chemistry. Your blood doesn't lie and imbalances showing up are all linked to something. How you feel can shift the blood chemistry. Dr. Bruce Berkowsky, N.M.D., M.H., H.M.C. has also done extensive research and education about in-depth organ associations to soul-level disharmony.

- Liver: Organ of heat, detoxification, anger (excess) and depression (deficient). Eliminates toxins allowing nutrients to enter.
  - Cooling and febrifuge essential oils: bergamot, helichrysum, lavender, orange, peppermint, Roman chamomile, rose and ylang ylang. *[handwritten: reduce fever]*

- Gallbladder: Organ where bile neutralizes acidity, emulsifies fat and is a "sweetener" to the body. It manifests bitterness, resentment, bold and impudent behavior, especially when someone has the "gall" to confront you or invade your boundaries.
  - Cholagogue and antispasmodic essential oils: pink grapefruit, lemon, peppermint, Roman chamomile, rose and rosemary. *[handwritten: promotes discharge of bile-purging do unward]*

- Kidneys: Filtering organ to flush waste, balance minerals and pH. Emotions of fear, shame and guilt show up with disharmony.
  - Diuretic, diaphoretic and pH regulating essential oils: bergamot, eucalyptus, geranium, juniper, lemon, pine and pink grapefruit. *[handwritten: heavy sweating]*

- Heart: Organ of rhythm, balance and stillness. This is where we experience love, joy, rejection, heartbreak, rapid heartbeat, palpitations and blood pressure issues.
  - Anti-inflammatory and cardiotonic essential oils: black pepper, helichrysum, rose, rosemary and ylang ylang. *[handwritten: stimulant]*

- Lungs: Organ of respiration, grief and guilt. Allows oxygen to fill tissues and removes the wastes, while allowing us to feel like we have room to breathe.

- o Expectorant and decongestant essential oils: eucalyptus, frankincense, lavender, myrrh, pine, ravinsara and thyme.

- Spleen: Organ involved with immune function and the removal of defective red blood cells. We experience obsession, compulsion and addictive behaviors.
  - o Immune strengthening, antiviral and antibacterial essential oils: cinnamon, geranium, lemon, orange, oregano and thyme.

- Stomach: Organ of digestion, absorption, assimilation and elimination. We experience worry, excessive mental chatter and malabsorption (hard time digesting a situation). ↗ *releaves gas*
  - o Digestive, anti-inflammatory and carminative essential oils: black pepper, coriander, fennel, ginger, marjoram, peppermint and Roman chamomile.

- Bladder: Somebody annoying you and you have a hard time establishing boundaries. We experience fear, shame and guilt - physical manifestations show up more in the form of a heated spasm.
  - *Cause or induce sweating*
  - o Diuretic and sudorific essential oils: juniper, lemon, pine, pink grapefruit and sandalwood.

- Pancreas: Works with the gall bladder for digestion and elimination. Organ of blood sugar management and digestive enzyme production. Responsible for feelings of joy and the "sweetness" of life. New science shows an association between diabetic ulcers and the feeling of powerlessness *(http://www.ncbi.nlm.nih.gov/pubmed/25856218)*.
  - o Circulation and digestive essential oils: bergamot, cinnamon, coriander, geranium, lavender, lemon and pink grapefruit.

- Blood: Organ of fluid transportation, circulation, pH, love, joy, broken heartedness and self-worth.
  - o Anti-inflammatory and circulatory essential oils: black pepper, cypress, lemon, lime, rose and rosemary.

Aromatherapy for the Soul - Spiritual PhytoEssencing™
Let me begin by giving you the backstory behind Spiritual PhytoEssencing™. Dr. Bruce Berkowsky, N.M.D., M.H., H.M.C. is the founder and teacher of the Natural Health Science System™ which has developed since the 1990's from research and private practice. It includes the integration of traditional naturopathy, herbology, nutrition, homeopathy, massage and bodywork, aromatherapy,

constitutional iridology, anthroposophical (spiritual) science as well as East and West healing arts and sciences. He devoted himself to the study and practice of the art and science of natural healing – mind, body and soul. He constructed his unique and dynamic system of health creation from a synthesis of the complementary aspects noted above which led him to the development of Spiritual PhytoEssencing™ (SPE).

SPE employs individualized essential oil blends and homeopathic-style dilutions derived from those blends to effect deep soul-level healing, and is based upon a synthesis of his experience of using specific aspects of aromatherapy, herbal medicine, doctrine of signatures, physiology, anthroposophical medicine, classical homeopathy, traditional Chinese medicine, depth psychology, color therapy, gemstone healing and the Kabbalah. Using the various modalities, it matches essential oils to the archetypes to connect to the deepest level of the soul to magnify truth of the authentic self.

Dr. Berkowsky's work has been published in several journals, and he is world renowned for his work in natural health and emotional, soul-level healing. He furthermore founded the Vital Chi Skin Brushing System™ which can sustain or reestablish the skin's functional integrity and youthful glow. According to Dr. Berkowsky, the systems primary function includes respiration, excretion, blood and lymph circulation, immunity and the conduction of vital chi (*www.NaturalHealthScience.com*), all powerful tools for that impact the entire body. Dr. Berkowsky's lifelong work can be found in his *Materia Medica/Spiritualis of Essential Oils* which consists of over 110 essential oil chapters covering their complete profile, or "portrait". His systems are truly an integration of all cultures, sciences and arts, worldwide.

Spiritual PhytoEssencing™ is a special, in-depth system used to create customized aromatherapy combinations using essential oils for deep soul-level connection and healing. The formulation of an oil blend is meant to accurately reflect an individual's "soul print", in order to ameliorate soul-level disharmony. It is the key to help keep the soul moving in a positive, harmonizing direction. It engages and connects our genetic and learned constitutions which dictate how we respond and react to various situations. For example, some people are natural introverts, while others are natural extroverts.

SPE works backwards through layers of our personality to the beginning of our self...the origin, the root of the soul, our most innermost realm, our authentic self.

The soul is made up of archetypes and images, not something that is tangible. It recruits intellect, feelings and the senses to develop knowledge of, and ongoing connection with, the higher consciousness. Carl Jung, Swiss psychiatrist and psychotherapist who founded analytical psychology (individualism), introduced us to this concept of archetypes. These are collective unconscious patterns of behavior and a unique intangible construct of the soul that generates a characteristic pattern of perceptible emotional and physical expressions. These are derived from the infinite inventory of past experiences stored within the collective unconscious. In turn, these expressions emanate a tangible image or pattern of behavior, response and reaction. The blend's goal is to work upon these patterns, through the core issue that lies beneath the surface, our false or perceived self, which attempts to shelter and contain the weaknesses of the true self. In doing this, those who have "lost" themselves during their life, find a way back to the person they are, authentically. This allows the person to then operate and govern their behavior from a place of true self, rather than the fabricated one.

Every experience we endure in our life is a stepping stone to define who we are. When we are exposed to something, it is like a pebble in the barrel. At some point, if the barrel is not drained, or cleansed, the barrel, "runeth over", causing havoc on the mind, body and soul interactions and functions. Through feedback, reinforcement, judgement and discipline, people tend to conform to a personality that is expected of them, and/or to try and help them "fit in" to their perceived environment. When you act from this perceived self, nothing is real. It is by operating as your true self, you can then better connect with people, animals, plants and the universe. A SPE, soul level blend can help you return to yourself, and bring disharmonies into harmony, thus having personal understanding, acceptance, self-love and happiness.

Doctrine of Signatures

The Doctrine of Signatures was popularized in the 1600's with the writings of Jakob Böhme. He suggested that God marked objects with a sign, or "signature", for their intended purpose, and that a plants physical make-up can give insight to its medicinal purposes. If you look at it, a plants physiology resembles various parts of the body, which can then be associated in helping ailments connected to that part of the body. The "signature" can also extend to environments or specific geographical areas native to the plants.

In aromatherapy, the Doctrine of Signatures can help you interpret the features of a plant for further understanding such as shape, leaf, stem, flower or root design, growth pattern, texture, color and scent of the plant material. This will give you further insight to matching plants and essential oils with an individual to construct a soul blend. Its many characteristics will translate into aromatherapy formulations and uses such as the structure integrity (physical and emotional strength or weakness), relationship with a particular organ or body function (i.e., rhizomes are typically related to the intestines), how it protects itself such as thorns (helps a person set boundaries and avoid invasion) and how it functions under certain weather conditions (if it requires wet soil, the person needing this oil may need extra hydration for optimal body function). Cardamom for example, has upright shoots with alternating blade-like leaves with pointed tips. The blades and points give us an idea of protection and defense. Does someone need to be defended and protected? If so, cardamom might be a good essential oil choice for a blend.

Just as shape gives insight, the color of the flowers and leaves can too. Yellow flowers for example are historically related to sluggish bile, peace and harmony, thus gall bladder function and mind-body centering. When our body rids wastes, we are happier, less bitter and resentful and can move forward with joy, hence yellow for sunshine.

Paying attention to the growing conditions and environment can enlighten you to the type of person who can be helped from a particular oil. For example, a plant that needs moist, but well-drained soil will require much hydration, but does not thrive in "swampy" conditions. So translate that to your client who has "swampy" issues such as candida and eczema. They would benefit from oils derived from plants that need hydration but well-drained soil. Understanding a plant's soul nature can deepen your connection with the human soul.

Plant Family Descriptions

There are thousands of plant species with over 60 families such as *Compositae, Labiatae* and *Umbelliferae* that give rise to the majority of essential oils *(http://www.theplantlist.org)*. These families are important to guide you in understanding the plant's nature and their family "signature" which translates into spiritual, mental, emotional and physical comprehension of an essential oil's origin. Here are the families of the essential oils discussed in the book.

Annonaceae: Ylang ylang. Woody trees and shrubs that includes paw paw and soursop. These oils have a sense of beauty and contentment.

Betulaceae: Birch. Deciduous nut-bearing trees and shrubs.

Burseraceae: Elemi, frankincense, myrrh and palo santo. Sometimes referred to as the frankincense and myrrh family, known for its non-allergenic resin. These oils have a lot of depth and bring about great wisdom.

Cistaceae: Cistus. Small family of shrubs known for their beautiful flower coverage when in bloom.

Compositae (asteraceae): Chamomile (German, Roman), davana, goldenrod, helichrysum, inula, Tanacetum annuum, tarragon and yarrow. Sunflower, dandelion and daisy family. These oils offer a deep level nurturing and healing.

Cupressaceae: Blue cypress, cypress and juniper (*communis, virginiana*). Conifer family most noted for having the largest, tallest, and stoutest individual trees in the world, along with being the second longest lived species. These oils provide strength and stability.

Ericaceae: Ledum and wintergreen. Considered the blueberry or heather family.

Geraniaceae: Geranium. Flowering plant.

Hypericaceae: St. John's Wort.

Iridaceae: Orris root. Iris family that are perennial plants that grow erect with a bulb or rhizomes.

Labiatae (Lamiaceae): Sweet Basil, catnip, clary sage, hyssop, lavender, marjoram, melissa, monarda, oregano, patchouli, peppermint, rosemary, sage, savory, spearmint and thyme. Mint family. Flowering plant, frequently aromatic and commonly used as a culinary spice. Each oil in this family have "notable" personalities and are confident in who they are without being conceited.

Lauraceae: Bay laurel, camphor (white), cassia, cinnamon, ho leaf, may chang, ravinsara and rosewood. Laurel, avocado and cinnamon family. Evergreen shrubs and trees, that mainly grow in warm climates. These oils offer comfort, security and confidence.

Leguminoseae (Fabaceae): Balsam peru. Legume family. Flowering trees or shrubs recognized by its fruit (legumes).

Myrtaceae: Cajeput, clove, eucalyptus, myrtle, niaouli and tea tree. Myrtle family that have woody evergreen trees. These oils offer room to breathe, grow and develop without constraints.

Myristicaceae: Nutmeg. Trees typically have colored sap and essential oils are known for their antifungal and antimicrobial properties.

Oleaceae: Jasmine. Olive trees are included in this family. These oils are nurturing and motherly.

Orchidaceae: Vanilla. Orchid family, fragrant, flowering plants with over 30,000 species in the world.

Pinaceae: Cedar (atlas, himalayan), fir (balsam, douglas, himalayan, siberian, silver), pine and spruce. Pine family. Mostly evergreen trees and shrubs that include some conifers, and have cones. These oils are good for resilience comes to mind when I think about oils in this family.

Piperaceae: Pepper (black). Pepper family; kava is in this family.

Poaceae (Gramineae): Lemongrass, citronella, palmarosa and vetiver. Grass family. These oils offer protection for self, help to set boundaries and overcome exhaustion from over giving.

Rosaceae: Rose. Rose family. Mostly evergreen but some are deciduous. These oils represent beauty, inside and out.

Rutaceae: Bergamot, grapefruit, lemon, lime, neroli, orange (bitter, sweet), petitgrain and yuzu. Citrus family. Flowering and fruit bearing trees, shrubs and plants. These oils are uplifting, inspiring and restoring, especially when there is chronic stress on the mind and body.

Santalaceae: Sandalwood. Sandalwood family; partially parasitic on other plants.

Styracaceae: Benzoin. Flowering trees with decorative white flowers. These oils provide deep soul nourishment.

Umbelliferae (Apiaceae): Ammi visnaga, angelica, anise, carrot, celery seed, cilantro, coriander, dill, fennel, galbanum and parsley. These have a distinctive "umbel"-like a flower stalk. Known to possess furanocoumarins (photosensitivity). These oils are nutritive and restorative.

Usneaceae: Oakmoss. Fruitcose lichens. These oils are helpful with parasitic relationships *(http://www.snh.org.uk/pdfs/publications/naturallyscottish/lichens.pdf)*.

Valerianaceae: Spikenard. Herbaceous plants with strong, disagreeable scented foliage. These oils are grounding and sedating.

Violaceae: Violet. Violet and pansy family. These oils connect with our inner child.

Zingiberaceae: Cardamom, ginger and turmeric. Ginger family. Plants are rhizomatous and most noted for their anti-inflammatory and antispasmodic properties. These oils add spice to your life.

Scent Classifications

Each essential oil has a unique and distinct scent. Some are stronger in one category while others may be a mixture of several scent categories. Geranium for example is more strongly classified as a floral scent, while oregano is a combination of herbaceous, earthy and spicy. When you understand an essential oil's scent, it can help you better choose which essential oils to have your client test during your Olfactory Sensory Testing™ session and to match up with your blend's purpose (explained more in the Art of Blending section).

You may find other aromatherapists referring to scent classifications by various names or descriptions, but they all share in the same message. Peter Holmes, for example, describes scent classifications as Fragrant Energetics. In Aroma Acupoint Therapy, he integrates an oil's energetic properties based on their aromatic qualities (*http://www.snowlotus.org/about-aroma-acupoint-therapy-tm/*). Jeanne Rose *(2003 Seminar, The Aromatherapy Book, 1993)*, refers to these classifications as Vocabulary of Odor. She explains, "Experiencing the different odors, enhances and develops the olfactory senses to help one distinguish between scents". I find using these classifications will add value, context and texture to your blending while steering you through a person's superficial and entrenched emotions. This is how you confront, conquer and achieve emotional healing, one layer at a time.

As you read about each of the scent classes, grab your essential oils and smell the ones listed so you can establish and build your relationship with these oils. This practice exercise will help develop your keen sense of smell, while learning the difference in the oil scents and further enhancing your intuition when you formulate and blend.

Class	Scent	Essential Oils
Floral	Semi-sweet, heavy, euphoric	Rose, neroli, ylang ylang
Fruity	Sweet, light	Mandarin, orange
Citrus	Sweet, sharp, uplifting	Grapefruit, lemon
Green/Vegetative	Grass, clean, green	Basil, thyme
Woodsy	Earthy, woody, smoky	Fir, pine, spruce
Herbaceous	Fresh, green	Clary sage, peppermint
Camphoraceous	Medicinal, opening	Eucalyptus, tea tree
Spicy	Warm, pungent, sharp	Clove, cinnamon, nutmeg

Aromatherapy for Children, Elderly & Animals

Aromatherapy can provide great comfort, relief and relaxation for children, elders and animals. Their systems however, are more sensitive so a smaller dilution ratio, shorter frequency and extra caution and education should be considered. If we look at the head-heart-gut physiology, children, elderly and animals have similar issues, but some may manifest in diverse ways. For example, those with ADD tendencies in children, elders and animals may experience similar experiences such as less focus and concentration, insomnia and lack of completing tasks. However, children and animals typically may be excessively hyper and less obedient, whereas elders may have excessive anxiety and nervousness.

Children, elders and animals depend on others for help, support and socialization. It is the circle of life. Children depend on parents and then there comes a point when parents must depend on children. It is both rewarding and stressful at the same time, for everyone. Physical, mental and emotional health is challenged so it is important during these times to find "me" time to replenish, rejuvenate and refuel your mind and body. In our society, internationally, we are seeing more multi-generation households with sometimes three to four generations under one roof. According to AARP, the U.S. 65-plus population is expected to more than double to 92 million by 2060 *(http://www.aarp.org/home-family/friends-family/info-04-2013/three-generations-household-american-family.html)*. There are Elder Laws in just about every country that protect elders from neglect. For example, in China, their "Elder Rights Law" states that adult children "should never neglect or snub elderly people" and should visit their parents "often," even if they live far away. This is helpful to combat feelings of abandonment, loneliness and loss (of independence and strength). France has a similar Elder Law. In Mediterranean and Latin cultures, taking care of elders is a common part of life, sharing responsibilities amongst the family. This is not only a great support system, but enhances socialization and decreases the amount of burden on one person. Common caretaking essential oils are Roman and blue chamomile, orange, vetiver and pine.

Mental: Head, Brain & Mind

With cognitive and brain functions, children and young animals are in an intense, upward learning curve, gaining new knowledge, sharpening problem solving abilities, rational thought processes, time management, memory enhancement and discipline just to name a few. Through their growth and development, a structured upbringing and classroom set-up can dictate their habits, actions, responses and behaviors via a type of conditioning. For example, learning and knowing right from wrong. Environmental structure along with the right nutrients, environment, habit reinforcement and social support, children can thrive in just about any situation or environment. Just watch when kids meet other kids for the first time, they just jump right in and start playing together. No judgement, just pure innocence. When there is a disruption in physical, mental and emotional balance, problems start appearing.

Some common concerns seen in children are behavior and cognitive responses such as ADD, ADHD, sensory disorders, learning abilities, Autism and emotional trauma. According to a KidSource study, it is conservatively estimated that 3 to 5% of the school-age population is affected by ADD. One in 110 children currently have Autism (www.autismspeaks.org) and one in seventy are boys. JennScents has created some aromatherapy blends for children expressing these issues and have seen an enhancement in performance and relaxation. I have found that Autistic children are very receptive and influenced by smells (http://atlanticinstitute.com/parp.html) and respond pretty quickly when exposed to diffused scents of *Cedrus atlantica*, lemon, vetiver, lavender and rosewood. It seems, children tend to respond quicker to aromatherapy than adults, especially when it comes to emotional healing. They typically respond within a few weeks rather than several months or years. They have less judgement, thought interference and resistance to the scents shifting their physiology into a positive state.

Children with mental and emotional challenges can do well when scents are diffused in the morning when they wake up to calm their demeanor, and before bed to help promote a restful sleep. Also, using it during the day to enhance cognition or calm nerves can be helpful. I have found frankincense to be helpful with bedwetting issues approximately 80% of the time (and even better results are experienced when combined with an herbal supplement or tincture of cornsilk).

With elders, because physiological body processes change and decrease with age, it becomes harder for cognitive and motor functions to operate at the same level and speed as younger generations. There is a decrease in metabolism of nutrients, vitamins, stomach acids and neurotransmission thus less memory, mobility and head-heart-gut communication. This can lead to depression, anxiety, fear, bitterness and resentment. When we are sad, our immune system is suppressed by over 50% *(Frey WH 2nd, DeSota-Johnson D, Hoffman C, McCall JT., "Effect of stimulus on the chemical composition of human tears," American Journal of Ophthalmology, 92:559-567, 1981.)*, which compromising the integrity of our body's abilities to combat foreign invaders. Scents can bring comfort, acceptance, understanding and peace to an elder, as well as encourage enhanced cognitive functions.

As we age, it is important to engage in a variety of brain exercises whether learning a new language or skill, memory word puzzles and engaging in conversation with recollections of past and present events. It is said that this continuous exercise of learning new information helps neurogenesis, the creation of new neurons in the brain, keeping cognition active and efficient *(http://www.ncbi.nlm.nih.gov/pmc/articles/PMC3264739/)*. Learning Tai chi is a perfect example, and coupling this with rosemary and lemon can assist as well. Because many cognitive processes run slower in mature brains than in children, more time and focus is needed to conquer a task. Memory recall is also affected greatly. So combining scents for concentration, focus and memory recall (fornix) specific essential oils would be beneficial. Changing their scent often would engage different parts of the brain and involve various parts of the body, creating circulation and movement between the head-heart-gut circuits.

Memory Booster: rosemary (verbenone), citrus, jasmine, peppermint

Mood Enhancer: citrus, cinnamon, sandalwood, basil,

Relax My Child: Roman chamomile, lavender and red mandarin

Study Buddy: Rosemary, lemon, jasmine, mints

Emotional: Heart (Feeling Center)
The heart and emotional physiology in kids, elders and animals allow them experience the same emotions…anger, grief, sad, lonely, fear, independence and so on. The difference is the wisdom (mental training) one has at that moment in time to respond to those emotions. Elders certainly have had a lifetime of trials and tribulations, practice and experience to respond differently than children and animals. Elders may become more numb or immune to the loss of something, more so than children, because they have experienced loss more. Children may react by crying and pitching a tantrum as they aren't familiar with something being taken away from them. They are used to a "taking" phase rather than a "giving" phase. Keeping the circulatory system moving via movement and exercise, physically and mentally, is highly beneficial for heart health but also to reduce emotional stuckness and immobility.

When children are confronted with a situation they have never experienced before, they don't really know how to respond yet. Some children may cry and become fearful. Others may well up with anger and become defensive or physically abusive. We typically see this behavioral response over time develop into a bullying mentality. They feel in order to boast their own self-confidence, they must put another down. Either way, these range of emotions are foundations for how these children will respond as they get older. If their responses are not properly addressed, it can lead to traumatic and debilitating circumstances. Thus, aromatherapy can be beneficial at every age to promote a positive self-image. Typically, responses are learned from either family, friends, television, movies and/or video games. All children know is that their heart wants what it wants and when they can't have it, an excessive or deficient emotion will rise. When we get older, the rational side steps in to calm those yearning heart feelings, allowing us to have a more controlled, sensible and balanced response. Our head and judgement steps in to prevail over our heart. We see it often, some children and young animals are shy and timid. Through social reinforcement and conditioning, they can learn self-confidence and esteem in a positive environment. When they are bullied, put down or hindered from reaching their potential, they began their development of negative perceptions about themselves, thus enhancing their low self-confidence and esteem. During adulthood, most people tend to "find their way", become comfortable with themselves and exhibit independence and confidence. We feel strongest and at our best. Then, as we enter into the elder years, we regress back into shy, timid, lack of self-confidence again because it is harder to keep the same momentum as in our younger years. Aromatherapy can help enter into childhood, graduate to adulthood and pass the baton to the next generation. Citrus scents are always uplifting for emotional balance. Woods and herbs are grounding to help us feel connected to ourselves and others. Florals and camphor's allow us room to breathe and manage stress.

> *Mind Over Body:* Orange, lime, pine, spearmint, fennel, frankincense
>
> *No More Nerves*: Bergamot, pink grapefruit, cinnamon, lavender
>
> *Nightmares, Night Fright, Fear:* Frankincense, patchouli (frequent nightmares may be related to parasitic activity)
>
> *Sleeping Sheep*: Frankincense, patchouli, lavender, ravinsara, orange

Physical: Gut (Action Center)
When it comes to our gut instincts and physical body, as children and baby

animals grow, their systems get stronger to support their growth spurts, puberty and overall health as they are exposed to different environments. Their experiences help them develop gut instincts and behavioral responses. Their energy levels are high and bodies more flexible for movement and exercise. Their body's just have an innate instinct of what to do. As our body ages for humans and animals, this focus shifts into maintaining the body, like keeping strong muscles and bones, exercising memory and providing nourishment for optimal immune function. Nutrition plays a huge role in all of this growth, development and maintenance. With lack of calcium, magnesium and vitamin D, it has been shown that bones and muscles are compromised. Children may break bones playing around. Elders may lose their balance and fall, breaking a limb or hip. Young animals such as puppies and kittens are very agile, flexible and energetic, while elder pets have a harder time jumping, getting up and down, running and having excessive energy.

Bum Balm: Roman Chamomile, lavender, myrrh, tea tree

Colds, flu, Congestion: Frankincense, eucalyptus, rosemary, spearmint

Skin Strengthener: Carrot, myrrh, frankincense, cypress, helichrysum

Tame the Tummy: Roman chamomile, peppermint, marjoram, fennel

Animals

Scent is how animals interpret the world. If you observe animals, they are always sniffing to investigate their surroundings. So it's no surprise that aromatherapy can be beneficial for animals, when used in a safe, educated and appropriate manner. Humans and most animals have similar olfactory systems, however there are two noticeable differences. One is the number of receptors, which is responsible for odor detection. Animals have up to 40-50 times more receptors than humans, giving them larger scent analyzing ability, thus making them more sensitive to smells. Dogs for example have 250-300 million receptors, horses have up to 100 million and cats have 200 million, compared to humans which have six million *(https://kmblog.kriticalmass.com/dogs-can-smell-cancer-on-your-breath/)*. The second difference is that a dog's brain devotes about 40 times greater scent processing ability than humans *(http://www.pbs.org/wgbh/nova/nature/dogs-sense-of-smell.html)*.

Animals, have a heightened sense of smell, detecting scents up to 10,000 times greater than humans, therefore less sensory stimuli the needed. This means that when you create formulas for animals, a smaller dilution ratio is required. When applying aromatherapy to animals, you will need to customize your blends based on the animal, size and weight *(http://www.dummies.com/how-to/content/understanding-a-dogs-sense-of-smell.html)*.

Dogs, horses, goats, pigs and llamas, for example, can be classified together, however adjust the potency and amount of scent exposure to match their weight, size and sometimes breed. Bloodhound and Basset Hound dogs are the most scent sensitive of dogs with over 300 million receptors, and commonly used to track scents for missing persons, drugs and even cancer *(http://dogtime.com/dog-health/general/18724-10-dog-breeds-with-the-best-sense-of-smell)*. Dogs have three times larger olfactory bulbs than humans. Even though horses and llamas are larger physically than dogs, their systems have similar sensitivities so more is not better. It actually can cause a toxic overload.

When conducting Olfactory Sensory Testing™ with horses, keep in mind that they have two olfactory bulbs, one on the left and one on the right. Each nostril is linked to its respectful side, so have them smell the scent per nostril. When they lean in, or smile, this tells us they like the scent. When they pull away, turn their nose up or run away, this would be a "no".

When using aromatherapy with animals, follow the safety precautions and continuously educate yourself. Animals can certainly benefit on a physical, mental and emotional level with aromatherapy. They are sensitive to changes, scents and the energy surrounding them. According to Kelly Holland-Azarro, RA, CCAP, CBFP, LMT, "Animals can experience many of the same emotions that humans do, as well as their own set of feelings and physical symptoms."

Here are some helpful essential oils for common issues. Remember to include your essential oils in a carrier before applying to an animal topically. You can also integrate or use hydrosols, as they offer great benefits and are gentler on their olfactory systems.

> *Aroma Flea Spray*: Eucalyptus, thyme, tea tree, rosemary, citronella
>
> *Obedience*: Rosemary, lemon, orange, basil
>
> *Skin Irritation*: Myrrh, patchouli, lavender, tea tree, bergamot
>
> *Fright (thunderstorms, fireworks)*: Roman chamomile, lavender, frankincense, jasmine, orange

Cats and guinea pigs are even more sensitive than dogs and horses. They should only be exposed to small amounts of scents for a very short periods of time (for example, 10-15 minutes at a time, only once or twice a day). Their olfactory system is not only more sensitive, but their excretory organs, especially their kidneys, cannot handle the strength and volume of scent chemical components. This means their bodies have a harder time metabolizing and effectively eliminating the chemical constituents that make up an essential oil(s). They can become intoxicated with high exposure and may stumble around and become very lethargic. These are signs of toxicity. Do not place aromas near the litter box or where they curl up to sleep. With these animals, you have to be more attentive and cautious when using aromatherapy.

> *Cat or Guinea Pig Wash*: Lavender, myrrh
>
> *Moody Blues*: Geranium, frankincense, ylang ylang, rose, bergamot
>
> *Social Butterfly*: Bergamot, peppermint, grapefruit, cinnamon

Fish and birds are incredibly more sensitive than cats, so it is recommended that you cover their cage and tanks before emitting scents in the surrounding air. Their bodies have a much harder time excreting the essential oil chemical constituents, greater than cats. I do not recommend aromatherapy exposure with these types of animals.

Although there are differences between children, elder and animal cognitive, social, motor and speech skills, the holistic remedies and essential oils will be the same. A recap of some specific safety measures are:

- Keep bottles out of the reach of children, animals and those with dementia.
- Dilute essential oils in a fat based carrier to help with the excretion process of their urinary system.
- Avoid over exposure when using an ultrasonic or plug-in diffuser, room sprays, cleaning products and ailment specific lotions. If an animal walks away from a scent being diffused, it's time to unplug it.

Aromatherapy & Complementary Holistic Health Modalities

Natural healing is not a new practice, but rather an ancient one. In European cultures, it is part of their standard common practice, however, not as much in western medicine. We are seeing a significant influx though in supporting science and thus the medical world is beginning to embrace this science-based "alternative" medicine in their own practices. I foresee many insurance companies broadening their coverage to include a variety natural health measures in their "preventive and reactive care" plans.

Aromatherapy is just one of many modalities in the realm of natural health. It engages the sense of smell, but also offers benefits to the other 4 senses – sight, touch, sound and taste. I'd like to throw in a 6th sense, called intuition. When combined with other complementary disciplines, together, they integrate, interconnect and heighten wellness to bring harmony and balance within the body and mind. Here are a few common natural health modalities:

Ayurveda	Flower Essences
Biofeedback	Homeopathy
Chakra/Energy Balance	Massage & Bodywork
Chiropractic	Meditation & Guided Imagery
Exercise, Tai Chi, Yoga	Traditional Chinese Medicine
Zumba	Acupuncture

My personal journey in natural health began in the late 1990's. I had several health issues including frequent respiratory and urinary infections, migraines, hormone imbalances and skin issues. I had a very paper intensive and time demanding career that left no time to be sick. Over the Thanksgiving and Christmas holiday season in 1999, I became very ill from taking two prescriptions for a urinary tract infection. This caused a severe reaction and antibiotic induced colitis (pseudomembranous colitis), Crohn's Disease and Irritable Bowel Syndrome (IBS). My life forever changed after this. I did several years of steroids and other anti-inflammatory, anti-depressant and pain medications, and eventually my body and mind was wiped out. It wasn't responding favorably, I was wasting away and just couldn't function – physically, mentally, emotionally or spiritually. I was a complete mess. My sister encouraged me to visit a local herb shop to see if there was anything "natural" that would give me some relief from the intestinal cramping, headaches, mental deficiencies and wasting condition. I met with the herbalist, Wendimere Reilly, and we had a great conversation about being educated and taking responsibility for my own health. We discussed how body processes work and its effects such as stress and elimination, and she taught me about the immense benefits of probiotics and essential oils. I chose to take a probiotic, which had also been recommended by my medical doctor. She also showed me how to make up an "Intestinal Soother" with Roman Chamomile essential oil and apricot seed oil (my very first essential oil lesson). I have to say, I was reluctant and skeptical but that very night, when my intestinal cramps flared up, as they usually did, I applied the Intestinal Soother and I couldn't believe that in minutes, the cramping started to subside. I know Roman chamomile is powerful, but there is science to prove it possesses anti-inflammatory properties *(http://www.ncbi.nlm.nih.gov/pubmed/21042790)*. For the first time in several years, I felt a glimpse of hope that I might survive this health crisis.

My lack of health almost cost me my life, but thankfully, I was able to learn about natural health remedies, and choose what was right for me. I found a doctor willing to help me integrate herbal, aromatherapy and medical therapies. I had to leave my work career that I really did love, as "healing Jennifer" became my new career. This journey introduced me to some incredible, knowledgeable and brilliant natural health practitioners and human beings. It also gave me the wisdom, courage and strength to begin JennScents, Inc. in 2002. Although this health journey was exhausting, life-altering, hard, tough and gut-wrenching, the beauty that came out of such tragedy was worth it. I am honored that I am here to pay my life lessons forward and inspire, encourage and empower others to fight for themselves. I now lead with the motto, "may you never know the disease you prevented", shared with me by my friend Dr. Jay Vanden Heuval.

Ayurveda Medicine
Ayurveda, meaning "the science of life" is a 5,000 year-old natural health system of Indian and Tibetan medicine. It is said to originate from the Indus Valley culture which is known for its practicalism. This culture believed in circulating resources among the living people rather than preserve them in temples or underground burials for the dead. They appeared to have a peaceful society. Human bones that were excavated did not show any signs of violence or battle wounds *(Melanie Sachs, http://www.diamondwayayurveda.com/)*.

Ayurveda intimately connects the mind, body and spirit for optimum health and well-being. It uses three Doshas, or categories of disharmonies or impurities - Vata, Pitta and Kapha. Ayurveda says that these doshas are responsible for maintaining balance in our environment, body, mind and spirit, simultaneously through healthy habits such as nutrition, hydration, lifestyle and herbal remedies. We each possess all three dosha characteristics, but in different proportions that construct our uniqueness. When balanced, there is a healthy state. When imbalanced, there is a disease state *(http://www.chopra.com/our-services/ayurveda)*.

Vata is related to our ability and pace of movement within our mind and body. It encompasses our central nervous system, joints, circulation and breathing. It is seated in the colon. When balanced, there is creativity, energetic vitality and enthusiasm. Imbalances are exhibited with fear, anxiety, attachment challenges and feeling unsettled. Pitta is related to our transformative processes, the body's metabolic and glandular systems, and is seated in our small intestines. When balanced there is concentration, decisiveness, intellect, ambition and discipline. Imbalanced, there is anger, malabsorption issues and fear that you are not good enough. Kapha is related to our physical nature, growth, development and hydration levels. It encompasses our tissues and structure, is seated in our stomach and supplies water to the entire body, moisturizes skin and preserves immunity. When balanced, there is love, forgiveness, nurturing and stability. Imbalanced, there is difficulty of letting go, insecurity, resentment and sluggishness *(http://umm.edu/health/medical/altmed/treatment/ayurveda)*.

In acupuncture, a Chinese originated therapy, there are meridian points that access certain pathways to enhance biochemical communications. In Ayurveda, there are marma points all over our body that are focused on releasing energy blocks in the mind and body to bring harmony and well-being. It is a part of the Chakra system. According to Melanie Sachs, at the 2014 NAHA World of Aromatherapy Conference, "If you anoint the body with right essential oils, you can balance subtle energies in minutes."

Chakras

Chakra is a Sanskrit word meaning "wheel or whirlpool", like a rotating wheel creating a spiraling intermingling of energies. There are seven Chakras which are described to be inter-connected power centers in the human body in which energy flows. Each chakra is associated with a particular part of the body and organs in which it provides the necessary energy to function. When an energy center is blocked, physiological and psychological imbalances occur. Similar to the process of the digestive systems, chakras receive, digest, assimilate, absorb and express vital force, or chi. Balanced chakras are influenced by our body shape and position, glandular processes, physical ailments, thoughts, behaviors, emotions and environment *(http://www.mindbodygreen.com/0-91/The-7-Chakras-for-Beginners.html)*.

7th Chakra: Crown (color is purple)

Represents complete openness to the divine light. It gives the ability to connect and build a relationship with spirituality. It is located at the tippy top of the head. It offers awareness and rational consciousness to our higher soul. When blocked, we may be close-minded and disconnection between our head, heart. It is associated with the brain, cerebral cortex, pituitary and pineal glands, hypothalamus and entire nervous system.

6th Chakra: Third Eye (color is blue)
Represents intuition, wisdom and intellect. It allows us to be open and see the big picture in its entirety. It is located on the forehead, between the eyebrows, just above the bridge of the nose. It offers understanding, knowledge, insight, inspiration, imagination and thought. When blocked, we may experience stuckness, not able to see the vision with clarity and exaggerated illusions. It includes the eyes.

5th Chakra: Throat (color turquoise)
Represents our ability to communicate, listen (hear) and express ourselves. It is located in the throat region, around the Adam's apple. It offers the ability to speak up for ourselves, express verbal and non-verbal communication effectively and realize purpose in life. When blocked, we may experience excessive talking, excessive shyness, fear of public speaking and inability to listen to others. It includes the throat, ears, mouth and hands.

4th Chakra: Heart (color is green)
Represents love, joy and inner peace. It is located in the center of the chest, just above heart. It supports circulation, respiration, peace, harmony, compassion, community, acceptance and forgiveness. When blocked, we may experience grief, rejection, abandonment, jealous, isolated and hold grudges. It includes the lungs and heart.

3rd Chakra: Solar Plexus (color is yellow)
Represents the ability to move forward with confidence, control and personal power, both mindfully and effectively. It is located upper abdomen in the stomach area. It offers metabolism, digestion and willpower. When blocked, we may experience anger, excessive control, lack of self-worth, low self-esteem, helplessness and lack of direction. It includes the stomach, gall bladder, liver and pancreas.

2nd Chakra: Sacral (color is orange)
Represents our ability to accept ourselves and others, and invite new experiences in. It is located in the lower abdomen region, about 2 inches below the navel and 2 inches in. It offers pleasure, passion, emotions, sexuality, creativity and energizes functions of assimilation of nutrients. When blocked, we may not be able to connect or relate with others, have a dependent and/or co-

dependent relationship, overindulge or lack of sexual desire. It includes the uterus, ovaries and testes.

1st Chakra: Root (color is red)
Represents our foundation and keeps us grounded. It is located at the base of the spine, in the tailbone region. It offers vital force, stability, security, survival, trust and a deep relationship with the natural world. When blocked, we may experience emotions of fear, negative, insecure and paranoia. It includes the kidneys, bladder and spine.

Flower Essences
Dr. Edward Bach, an English physician developed flower essence remedies in the 1930's. He was a homeopath, bacteriologist and pathologist that focused original research on vaccines. One day in 1917 when Dr. Bach was treating injured soldiers returning from France, he collapsed and suffered a life-threatening hemorrhage. His fellow colleagues operated on him to remove a tumor and diagnosed him with three months live. He died 20 years later, but not before aspiring to discover a more holistic approach in medicine. Throughout these 20 years, he was steadfast in learning about thousands of plants in nature and used his intuition as guidance to choose 38 specific ones that were associated with a basic human emotion. According to the Bach Centre *(http://www.bachcentre.com/centre/drbach.htm)*, "He found that when he treated the personalities and feelings of his patients, their unhappiness and physical distress would be alleviated naturally as the healing potential in their bodies was unblocked and allowed to work once more."

Richard Katz founded the Flower Essence Society (FES), a non-profit organization, in 1979. He and his wife, Patricia Kaminski, continued to expand Dr. Bach's work creating additional 100+ flower essences. They also authored the *Flower Essence Repertory* (2004). The premise is that the essence of a flower, at its true core nature, resonates and awakens something within us to exert mind, body and soul empowered development. Dr. Bach said, "*Disease is in essence the result of conflict between soul and mind. So long as our souls and personalities are in harmony, all is joy and peace, happiness and health. It is when our personalities are led astray from the path laid down by the soul, either by our own worldly desires or by the persuasion of others that a conflict arises.*"

A flower essence is a liquid preparation created by immersing a flower into water and exposing the preparation to sunlight or heat. This infuses the preparation with healing properties from the life energy and spiritual elements contained in the flower. Flower remedies are made from these flower preparations (essences), and employed to help address, shift, change and influence emotional concerns on a deeper soul and spiritual level.

Flower essences differ from essential oils, in that it's not the chemical constituents creating the shifts, but instead, it is the life forces contained within the water-based matrix of the plant. Flower essences are energetic imprints of the life force of plants which interact with our human bodies, and spark specific qualities within us. Flower Essences are typically safe when integrated with traditional and alternative medicine. They are most commonly taken orally from a dropper bottle directly under the tongue, or in some water. They are effective in topical application such as skin crème, bath salts and massage oil.

I began to personally use flower essences around 2002. The Bach Rescue Remedy was one of my favorite as it helped with stage fright and my fear of public speaking. I noticed my nerves not freaking out as much, I didn't break out into a cold sweat and pass out, like I typically would do if I have to speak in front of a group of people. From this moment on, I was intrigued and a consumer for life. Most flower essences are based in a small amount of alcohol. If you don't do well with alcohol, or are a recovering alcoholic, there are a couple brands that are glycerin based. I found a Distress Remedy in glycerin that worked just as well as the Bach Rescue Remedy so that is my personal favorite.

As I experimented with flower essences personally, I had a thought, what if I added them to my aromatherapy blends? Would it enhance the psycho-spiritual affects complementary to my blend's purpose? I had a few customers that were excited to see how their mind and body would respond, so together, we chose which flower essences to integrate into their aromatherapy custom blend. The results were significant. Not only did the blend conquer the purpose we were striving to achieve, but it created a notable change within just a couple of days in their emotional and mental stability, strength and enthusiasm. So it has become a common practice for me to integrate flower essences and essential oils in my aromatherapy blends.

Homeopathy
Homeopathy is natural, non-toxic, small and highly diluted substances made from plant, mineral, metal, insect and other sources used to stimulate the body to create homeostasis – balance between physical, mental and emotional. The preparation is known as potentization, and consists of successive dilutions followed by shaking in ten hard strikes against an elastic body at each dilution stage. You continue this process until the desired potency is achieved. Ironically, the more it is diluted, the stronger the final product. This vigorous agitation

following each dilution is thought to transfer some of the "spiritual essence" of the substance to the water.

The origination of Homeopathy is credited to Dr. Samuel Hahnemann, a German doctor and chemist in 1796, however there is documentation dating back as early as Hippocrates in 400 B.C. It follows the Law of Similars, or "likes curing likes", meaning that if a specific substance can cause a healthy person to get sick from it, then that same substance can also help heal a person that is sick with it. Hahnemann believed the underlying causes of disease were occurrences that he termed *miasms*, and that homeopathic preparations addressed these. His homeopathic philosophy is also applied in Spiritual PhytoEssencing™.

Homeopathy follows the Law of Similars, but also believes in matching the complete homeopathy profile of the client to the complete profile of the remedy. They use the least amount of solution with just one homeopathic remedy at a time, rather than a combination of several remedies. Although, there are certain instances where homeopathic combinations are created to conquer a specific issue. When I integrate homeopathic dilutions in my aromatherapy blends, I just choose one *(www.nationalcenterforhomeopathy.org/)*.

So what role do they have on emotions? They can help to connect with certain emotions to help them move out or in to combat stagnation and lethargy. They activate the body's own natural ability to heal like spark plugs that ignite energy. They create a more powerful synergy that works on specific emotions, especially when married with essential oils.

A common question I hear is, "can you combine flower essences, homeopathy and essential oils?" Well, I personally do and find that I achieve greater, more precise and effective results. I follow the same essential oil dilution ratio chart and add by the drops (not droppers) of flower essences and homeopathics. The formula will depend on the client's current emotional status, sensitivity level and goals of the overall blend.

Massage and Bodywork
Massage and touch therapies have been around since ancient civilizations and was a part of their daily "health care" practices. Ayurveda incorporates it into their health system as one way to help someone re-establish harmony between themselves and their environment, thus enhancing their immune system *(http://www.ncbi.nlm.nih.gov/pubmed/15630807)*. Egyptian paintings depicted pictures of a person massaging another. The Chinese combined the philosophies of massage and Traditional Chinese Medicine to evolve such therapies as acupressure ad

acupuncture. The Greek used massage before athletic competitions to prepare their body for activity. The famous Greek physician, Hippocrates was credited with changing the direction of massage strokes toward the heart to enhance circulation and facilitate waste elimination. He suggests, "The way to health is to have an aromatic bath and scented massage every day." Galen, a Roman physician, used massage therapy for various physical injuries, enhance circulation and loosen up joints and muscles. Fast forward to the 1950's, and Marguerite Maury, a French biochemist, was credited for integrating and utilizing essential oils in massage oils for dermal applications, hence the popularity of Aromatherapy Massage *(http://umm.edu/health/medical/altmed/treatment/massage)*.

Today, there is longstanding history and scientific studies proving its efficacy for pain relief, muscle tension, relaxation, mental health and much more. It truly is a mind-body-soul therapy, contrary to some beliefs that it is just a luxury. It's not just for athletes and the wealthy, but for anyone and everyone needing relief from stress, pain, tension, overworked muscles and human touch, both humans and animals. It is very beneficial on an emotional and mental level to help one connect energetically with another, especially during times of grief, guilt, anger and loneliness. We are seeing it integrated into many medical facilities as well as day spas, chiropractic and dental offices, grocery stores and other businesses.

There is a standard of practice among licensed massage and body work therapist. One must conduct themselves and maintain legal, ethical, professional and confidential business practices at all times. They must honor their roles and establish professional boundaries with clients as well as employ proper and responsible applications *(http://www.ncbtmb.org/standards-practice)*. Each state has their own Code of Ethics connected to licensure, but there are also "universal" guidelines of respect.

Massage is a "hands on" treatment in which a trained and licensed therapist manipulates muscles and other soft tissues of the body to improve circulation, overall health, enhanced digestion and elimination *(http://www.ncbi.nlm.nih.gov/pubmed/26099205)*, pain relief and so much more *(http://www.ncbi.nlm.nih.gov/pubmed/25808188)*. Examples are Swedish (developed in 1800's by a Swedish doctor and introduced in the US in the 1850's), Deep Tissue (more detailed body work on specific muscle groups), Neuromuscular, Trigger Point (tender spots on injured muscles), Thai (deep massage techniques coupled with stretching *[http://www.ncbi.nlm.nih.gov/pubmed/25682523]*), Sports, Shiatsu (raising energy levels so body can naturally enhance organ functions to resist invaders *[http://www.ncbi.nlm.nih.gov/pubmed/25489534]*), Reflexology (discovery credited to the Egyptians), Pregnancy and Pediatric just to name the most popular.

59

Acupressure uses precise finger placement and pressure over meridians, specific points along the body to offer relief from pain and stress and to facilitate the body's own healing processes during times of disharmony.

Body Treatments
Body treatments often employ an apparatus such as an exfoliating cloth, hot stones, body brush and/or herbal wrap to exfoliate and hydrate the skin, removing dead skin cells to encourage healthy cell proliferation and rejuvenation.

Craniosacral is a light, gentle touch technique that works deep throughout the body to relieve tension and free restrictions including the central nervous system. This gentle approach allows the body to self-correct and release unwanted stress and pain allowing for a greater sense of well-being, relaxation and to restore circulatory flow.

Lymphatic Drainage is a light touch technique using rhythmic strokes to stimulate, cleanse and drain the lymphatic system and surrounding tissues. It is beneficial for puffiness, swelling, congestion and overall fatigue *(http://www.ncbi.nlm.nih.gov/pubmed/21523925)*.

'M' Technique® was founded and developed by Jane Buckle, Ph.D., R.N. as a method of gentle, structured touch for the critically ill and fragile. Jane has a background in critical care nursing, massage therapy, clinical aromatherapy and herbal and aromatic medicine and developed this for caregivers, family members, volunteers, patient ambassadors and friends as well as nurses and other health professionals *(http://www.rjbuckle.com/)*.

Reiki is a Japanese technique placing hands lightly on or above the body used for stress reduction and relaxation. This enables the body to strengthen the body's vital force, facilitating its own restoration from disharmony *(https://nccih.nih.gov/health/reiki/introduction.htm)*.

Reflexology is a light touch technique on the hands and feet used to stimulate various organs and body systems, proving beneficial for overall well-being, fatigue, cognitive functions, anxiety and pain *(http://www.ncbi.nlm.nih.gov/pubmed/23730858)*.

Traditional Chinese Medicine (TCM)
Traditional Chinese Medicine (TCM) is a holistic health system developed over 2,500 years ago that integrates nutrition, herbs, massage, acupuncture,

bodywork and environmental balance to gain and maintain health. The focus is not on symptoms we experience, which is common in Western Medicine, but rather looks at why symptoms are occurring in the first place. It addresses the root cause of disharmony by examining excess and deficient tissue states. They further employ a 5 element approach when assessing imbalances in the body as well as focus on interconnections between mind, body and spirit.

In TCM, they refer to our vital or universal energy as Chi. This is a unifying flow of energy of living and non-living matter that activates the "electricity" within our being, thus generating physical energy for overall mind and body functions. Chi travels via 12 major sets of meridians (12 on the right and 12 on the left), which is a network of interconnecting pathways throughout the entire body. Each pair of meridians are associated with a specific organ or function and cycle every 24-hours. These are used in the practice of acupuncture to harmonize the disharmonies.

TCM seeks harmony between duel opposites but balancing and interdependent forces called *yin* and *yang*. Yin and Yang together, like two halves to a puzzle, create wholeness and the ultimate harmony. The yin force is the black part of the yin-yang symbol. It is related to female energy, introverted, rest, contraction, cold, dampness and internal organs. The yang force is the white part of the yin-yang symbol. It is related to male energy, extroverted, energy and activity, expansion, hot, dryness and exterior of the body (skin and muscles). The two small circles in each yin and yang portion represents a little of the opposite force within one another. Yang is flowing into and creating yin and vice versa on a continuous, rotating cycle.

Another component of TCM is the five element model which consists of wood, fire, earth, metal and water. It demonstrates the interdependent relationships and responses between the human body and the natural environment. Deficiencies and excesses in these elements can help identify health and sickness. Wood burns via Fire, which turns into the earth. The earth, in its densest form is metals, which then influenced by water. Water nourishes wood, and the cycle continues, just like the hands on a clock. There should be constant movement among the elements, not allowing for us to be stagnant or stuck in one place for too long, but rather cycling through the phases optimally.

The first of the elements is Wood and includes liver and gall bladder. When in excess, or vented, there may be emotions and physical manifestations of anger, frustration and irritation. When deficient, or suppressed, there may be depressed, despondent, feel defeated and have deep-seated bitterness.

The fire element includes the heart and small intestines. When in excess, there may be extreme excitement and laughter, nervous spasms such as anxiety, jumpy and uneasiness. When deficient, there may be boredom, feeling uninterested, humorless, coldness and just burned-out.

The earth element includes the stomach, pancreas and spleen. When in excess, there may be sympathy, concern, compassion, worry and over-protectiveness. When deficient, there may be constant complaining, cantankerous, feelings of neglect and not able to easily adjust to new things and surroundings.

The metal element includes the lungs and large intestines. When in excess, there may be grief, sadness, feeling hurt and smothered without room to breathe. When deficient, one can be insensitive, uncaring, defensive and rebellious.

The water element includes the kidneys and bladder. When in excess there may be fear, shyness, scared, indecisive and a lack of will-power. When deficient, one may feel like they have to struggle for power, success and social standing.

In Spiritual PhytoEssencing™, Dr. Berkowsky developed a six element model. This model was inspired by the Chinese five element model, but does not replace it. Rather, it is an evolution from it that was created to match the specific uniqueness necessary in deep soul level healing. It also was influenced by anthroposophical medicine, the Kabbalah, the yogic chakra system and Native American spiritual understanding. There are two main differences. One is with the Fire Element which has been divided into Light and Warmth. Additionally, Metal is one the primary elements in the Chinese Five Element Theory, with Air considered to be a component of Metal. In the Six Element Paradigm, these are reversed and Air is considered to be a primary element with Metal to be a sub-element that is a hybrid of certain aspects of Air and Earth. Similarly to the Ayurveda five element philosophy of Air, Earth, Ether (light, life, consciousness, space), Fire and Water. Furthermore, with the adjustments made in the Six Element Paradigm, there are also some distinct differences in the classification of organ affinities. For instance, in the Chinese Five Element Theory, the thyroid gland is not considered at all. In the Six Element Paradigm, the thyroid gland is associated with both the Air and Warmth elements.

The six elements are Light, Water, Warmth, Air, Earth and Wood. This is explained in explicit detail in Dr. Berkowsky's *Six Element Paradigm Workbook* (*www.NaturalHealthScience.com*).

Essential Oil Profiles

Understanding a plant can give you great insight into an essential oils "personality", enabling you to use the properties, benefits and uses to choose an application method and blend formulation. I'll discuss 105 essential oils in great detail including scent and plant description, properties, extraction method, physical, mental and emotional benefits, chakras, history and contraindications (precautions). Keep in mind, if you have a true, genetic allergy to the plant, you should avoid use. Some environmentally and nutritionally induced allergies, can be overcome through achieving a healthier gut and emotional state.

References: *http://www.pfaf.org/user/plantsearch.aspx,* *Dr. Berkowsky Synthesis Materia Medica/Spiritualis of Essential Oils http://www.thewildclassroom.com/biodiversity/floweringplants/Intro.htm)*

I share the note category – top, middle and base. Notes are discussed in-depth in the Art of Blending Chapter. For now, notice that I have assigned each note a specific number to show you where its intensity falls on the "note spectrum". If I do not list a number next to the note, you can assume it is a solid, middle of the scale, note.

> ➤ **Top**: 1-3 (1 is the highest top note, 3 is a lower top note close to a high middle note)

> ➤ **Middle**: 4-7 (4 is the highest middle note [light], 7 is a lower middle note close to a high base note [heavier])

> ➤ **Base**: 8-10 (8 is the highest base note [lighter], 10 is a lower base note [heaviest])

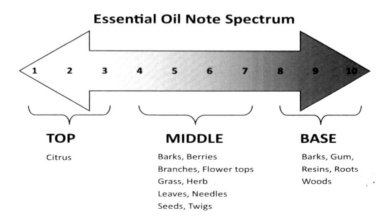

Essential Oil Note Spectrum

1 2 3 4 5 6 7 8 9 10

TOP
Citrus

MIDDLE
Barks, Berries
Branches, Flower tops
Grass, Herb
Leaves, Needles
Seeds, Twigs

BASE
Barks, Gum,
Resins, Roots
Woods

Ammi visnaga (*Ammi visnaga*)

Scent: Strong, earthy, herbaceous, green, slight musk with sweet undertones

Note: Middle to Base, 7-8, however 1 drop is very strong and can overtake a blend.

Extraction Method: Distillation

Parts Used: Blossom, plant, seed

Plant Description: Ammi is a flowering plant that can grow as tall as 3-4 feet, is commonly referred to khella, or the "toothpick plant". The leaves are edible and aromatic. It produces tiny white flowers, supported by toothpick-like pedicles, that when in bloom are grouped together in clusters, that sometimes look like an "umbrella shape". The seeds (commonly referred to as the fruit) have the shape of a tear drop and are used when dried. It prefers to grow in well-drained and slightly acidic soil in full to semi-shaded sunlight. It is in the Umbelliferae family.

Chemistry: Monoterpenes (sabinene, phellandrene, pinene); Esters (bornyl acetate, isoamyl 2-methyl butyrate, isopentyl isovalerate); Sesquiterpenes (germacrene); Furanochromone (khellin, visnagin, khellol, ammiol, visammiol, khellinone), Monoterpenols (linalool, terpineol, terpin-4-ol); Ketones (camphor, carvone); *(Phytochemistry and Medicinal Properties of Ammi visnaga (Apiacae). Saima Hashim, Asad Jan, Khan Bahadar Marwat and D Muhammad Azim Khan. Pak. J. Bot., 46(3): 861-867, 2014.)*

Main Body Systems: Circulatory, respiratory, urinary

Properties: Analgesic, antibacterial, antihistamine, anti-inflammatory, antispasmodic, antiviral, decongestant, diuretic, expectorant, lithotriptic, muscle relaxant and restorative.

Physical: Adrenal support, bladder spasms, cardiovascular circulation, cold and flu, dry cough, hormone balance, inflammation, muscle tension, soreness, muscle spasms, pan relief, respiratory issues (asthma, bronchitis, pneumonia), skin issues and vasodilative (headaches and heart).

Mental: Anxiety, creativity, dizziness, high strung, inner strength, lightheadedness, mental confusion, nervousness and stress.

Emotional: Agitation, annoyance, betrayal, bitterness, deep emotional trauma, fright (holds breathe when scared), grief, guilt, irritability, resentment, room to breathe, smothered and suffocated.

Chakra: 1st (root), 4th (heart), 5rd (throat)

History: Ammi is probably most noted to enhance breathing when respiratory concerns are present, and/or after exercise or rigorous activity, Used by many ancient cultures for pulmonary ailments. Egyptians used the seeds in a tea for kidney stones and bladder infections. Morocco used it for diabetes, heart and kidney issues.

Personal Experience: I personally have found this to be helpful with those who have severe lung or respiratory concerns, especially when there is long-term exposure to chemical cleaners and products (i.e., bleach), such as hairdressers, nail techs, mechanics, lawn maintenance workers, stay at home parents, housecleaners and commercial cleaners. Many people have reported that this long-term chemical exposure has affected and decreased their sense of smell. It seems the lining of the nasal passageway gets irritated and compromised, not allowing adequate scent molecules to be delivered optimally. I have had several friends regain their smell intensity after diffusing *Ammi visnaga* daily for at least 60-120 days (often combines with other culinary oils). On an emotional level, I have found it to be beneficial for deep-seated grief, significant loss and despair.

✳ **Contraindications**: Phototoxic and should avoid when taking blood thinners. ✳

Angelica *(Angelica archangelica)*

Scent: Herbaceous, curry-like with slight sweet, sour and musky undertones, opening

Note: Middle 6

Extraction Method: Steam distillation

Parts Used: Roots or seeds

Plant Description: This is a biennial plant that can grow up to 5-6 feet tall. It does not mature much in its first year. By the second year it flowers and completes its life cycle by the third year. When it blooms, typically in the summer, there are tiny white pale yellow or green flowers, clustered together in small groups almost like cotton. It is an aromatic plant, with strong stems, and medium sized serrated leaves. The seeds grow in late summer to early fall. It has long, spindle-shaped, thick roots. It prefers moist, acidic soil in an open semi-shaded area. It is very hardy and can tolerate severe frosts without damage. It is in the Umbelliferae family.

Properties: Analgesic, antibacterial, antifungal, anti-inflammatory, antioxidant, antispasmodic, carminative, diaphoretic, diuretic, febrifuge, immune-stimulant, restorative and tonic.

Chemistry: Monoterpenes (camphene, cymene, limonene [*d*, *l*], myrcene, phellandrene, pinene, sabinene, ocimene); Sesquiterpene (bisabolene); Esters (bornyl acetate); Monoterenols (linalool); Lactones (2-angelicine, angelica lactone, bergaterpene [furanocoumarins]) *(http://www.ncbi.nlm.nih.gov/pubmed/24788027)*.

Main Body Systems: Circulation, glandular, urinary

Physical: Alopecia (hormone related), anemia, arthritis, blood purifier, candida, circulation, digestive aid (gas, bloating), female issues (PMS, hot flashes, moody), gout, inspires desire for intimacy, low blood sugar, lymphatic congestion, respiratory and intestinal inflammation and urinary concerns.

Mental: Anosmia, anxiety, articulation, deepens spiritual connection, exhaustion, fatigue, inner wisdom, insomnia, left-right brain balance, nervousness, strengthens ability to communicate, stress and worry.

Emotional: Bitterness, deep seated fear, grounding, emotional rollercoaster, PTSD, promotes a sense of spiritual protection, release negative thoughts, resentment, restores emotional balance, self-love and strengthens aura.

Chakra: 1st (root), 4th (heart), 7th (crown)

History: European cultures used angelica for many medicinal purposes as well in food dishes. Folklores shares that many cultures believe it to provide psychical protection and have a connection to the "angels". It has been connected with offering benefits from the 17th Century Great Plague, and was commonly grown on the grounds of monasteries where it was referred to as "Angel Grass." Indian tribes used as a restorative. Recent studies are showing its power to fight against mold, oxidative stress and as an insect repellent. In TCM it is known as Dong Quai, often referred to as the "female ginseng".

Personal Experience: I use this essential oil to enhance my connection to myself and spiritualty. It is as if it opens up a special passageway for me to feel whole, and complete. It has been great to reduce anxiety, promote mood stability and reduce stress related skin issues. I can breathe deeper and I feel less congested – physically, mentally, emotionally and spiritually.

 Contraindications: Phototoxic. Use caution during pregnancy due to its emmenagogue property. Use caution with diabetes, as it may increase blood sugar in urine.

Anise *(Pimpinella anisum)*

Scent: Licorice scented, sweet, hearty with herbal undertones

Note: Middle 7, however 1 drop can go a long way as it can overtake a blend.

Extraction Method: Steam distillation

Parts Used: Seeds and flowering tops

Plant Description: Also referred to as aniseed. It is a fragrant and mineral-rich, annual plant that can grow up to 2 feet high. It has thin stems with small feathery leaves and produces small, clusters of white flowers that sit on top of thin pedicles. It is very sensitive to frosts and may not survive in cold, damp temperatures, thus anise prefers warmth and sunlight in dry, well-drained, alkaline soil. It does need to be sheltered from the wind, as it doesn't do well if uprooted or transplanted. The brown seeds mature about one month after pollination. It flourishes well when grown near coriander. It is in the Umbelliferae family.

Properties: Analgesic, antibacterial, antidepressant, antispasmodic, antifungal, carminative, digestive, expectorant, galactagogue, hepatoprotective, insecticide, stimulant.

Chemistry: Ethers (trans-anethole, estragole, safrole); Monoterpenols (anisol, linalool, a-terpineol); Aldehydes (anisicaldehyde); Sesquiterpenes (α-himachalene); Coumarins and Ketones *(http://www.ncbi.nlm.nih.gov/pubmed/18266152)*.

Main Body Systems: Glandular, intestinal, nervous

Physical: Adrenal support, boost cellular energy, colds, cold extremities, colic, digestive aid, fever, halitosis, libido support, mouth sores, muscle pain, nausea, PMS, respiratory concerns and stimulates intestinal function.

Mental: Cognitive strength, concentration, exhaustion, fatigue, frozen in a situation, indecisive, memory recall, migraines, nervous and trouble adjusting to new circumstances.

Emotional: Accepting, anger, depression, emotionally cold, fear of failure, feel bogged down and overwhelmed, frustration, grief, guilt, repression and timid.

Chakra: 1st (root), 2nd (sacral), 3rd (solar plexus)

History: Often used to flavor culinary dishes. The Romans would add into desserts as a digestive aid. It has been used to scent the artificial rabbit used at greyhound races, since most dogs love the scent of anise. Hippocrates recommended it for coughs. Egyptians used it to remove excessive mucus from the lungs. Amazonians used for stomachaches in children. Iranian traditional medicine used as a carminative and galactagogue. Studies show that when combined with coriander, it may ward off bedbugs, lice and red spider mites.

Personal Experience: I use this essential oil to stimulate and enhance digestion, reduce gas, bloating, indigestion, acid reflux and silent reflux. It nourishes me during fatigue and exhaustion, especially when enduring a chronic stressful situation.

Contraindications: Galactagogue *(stimulates breast milk production).* Poisonous to pigeons.

Balsam, Peru (*Myroxylon balsamum var. pereirae*)

Scent: Rich, sweet, balsamic, vanilla-like scent with spicy undertones

Note: Base 9

Extraction Method: Steam Distillation

Parts Used: Resin

Plant Description: It is an evergreen tree that can grow to heights of 115 feet. The bright green, ovate leaves are shiny with a pointed tip. The flowers are pea-like with slender, fragrant racemes that produce long, slender yellow fruit (pods). It prefers shaded areas in tropical climates with moist but well-drained soil. It is a member of the Leguminoseae family.

Properties: Antibacterial, antifungal, anti-inflammatory, antiparasitic, antiseptic, antiviral, circulatory stimulant, expectorant, stimulant and vulnerary.

Chemistry: Esters (benzoic acid, cinnamic acid, benzyl benzoate); Sesquiterpenols (farnesol, nerolidol); Aldehydes (vanillin); and Coumarins.

Main Body Systems: Intestinal, respiratory, urinary

Physical: Asthma, bed sores, bronchitis, bruises, diaper rash, dry cough, gastro-intestinal issues, H. pylori, laryngitis, mastitis, respiratory concerns, rheumatism, skin issues (rashes, eczema, dry), stimulates low blood pressure and ulcers.

Mental: Adapt to changes, anxiety, communication, confidence, indecisive, discontent, distracted easily, finding purpose, meditation, mental blockages, mental clarity, mood swings, nervousness, stress and worry.

Emotional: Abuse, broken heart, emotional wounds, fear, feel beaten down, inner strength, let go of grudges, protect from toxic relationships, speaking up for self, strength to "hold it together", especially during trauma.

Chakra: 1st (root), 3rd (solar plexus), 4th (heart), 6th (third eye), 7th (crown)

History: The genus name means "sweet oil" or "perfume" (*Myro*) and "wood" (*xylon*). Its resin is a common food additive and flavoring in cough syrups, soft drinks and chewing gums. It is a popular fixative in perfumes and soaps. Historically was used medicinally for hemorrhoids, cough lozenges, surgical dressings and dental cement.

Personal Experience: I like to use this for dry cough, throat issues, GI spasms and skin irritations. Emotionally, it warms the heart, comforts the soul and grounds the spirit.

Contraindications: Skin irritant, may cause allergies.

Basil, Holy (*Ocimum sanctum*)

Scent: Herbaceous, sweet licorice, hearty green scent with slight spicy and camphor undertones

Note: Middle 6

Extraction Method: Steam Distillation

Parts Used: Leaves and flowering tops

Plant Description: Perennial herb that can grow up to 2 feet high. It has dark green leaves with purple veins, on strong, hairy stems. It produces dark purple flower stems with tiny white flowers. It grows well in warm, sunny weather in light but mineral-rich and well-drained soil. It is sensitive to cold temperatures and typically do not survive frosts. It is in the Labiatae family.

Properties: Adaptogen, analgesic, antibacterial, anti-depressant, antifungal, antiseptic, antispasmodic, antiviral, digestive, diuretic, emmenagogue, expectorant, febrifuge, hepatoprotective, insecticide, mucolytic, nervine and sudorific.

Chemistry: Phenols (eugenol); Ethers (estragole); Alcohols (linalool); Monoterpenes (camphene, cineole, carvacrol); Sesquiterpenes (caryophyllene, bisabolene); Triterpene (urosolic acid) *(http://www.ncbi.nlm.nih.gov/pmc/articles/PMC3249909/)*.

Main Body Systems: Circulatory, glandular, nervous, urinary

Physical: Adrenal fatigue, arthritis, circulation, constipation, cough (spastic), diarrhea, herpes, kidney support, nausea, nerve pain, paralysis, respiratory issues (bronchitis, asthma), ringworm and vein health.

Mental: Addictions, alertness, anxiety, confusion, courage, dementia, depression, energizing, exhaustion, frazzled nerves, headaches, memory, mental clarity, panic attacks, refreshes the mind, sharpens cognitive function, stress relief and uplifting.

Emotional: Assertiveness, bitterness, deepens spirituality connection, fear, inspire passion, feel attacked (by snake-like personalities), negativity, resentment, self-doubt, shame, self-worth and warms the heart.

Chakra: 1st (root), 2nd (sacral), 3rd (solar plexus), 4th (heart), 7th (crown)

History: In Sanskrit, the name of Holy Basil is Tulsi, meaning incomparable. Used for thousands of years in Ayurveda for its multitude of healing properties. Popular in India for religious and medicine purposes. In Egypt, leaves were scattered on graves of departed loved ones.

Personal Experience: I use holy basil to nourish and strengthen my nerves, adrenal function and circulation. It helps me manage my stress with a balanced focus and allows me to not feel overwhelmed or overburdened.

Contraindications: Noted as a mild skin irritant (more than other basils).

Basil, Sweet (*Ocimum basilicum*)

Scent: Herbaceous, green with bitter, sweet, spicy undertones

Note: Middle 5-6

Extraction Method: Steam Distillation

Parts Used: Leaves and flowering tops

Plant Description: Perennial herb that can grow up to 2 feet high. It has vibrant dark green ovate leaves on thin but sturdy stems. It produces dark purple flower stems with tiny white flowers. It grows the best in warm, sunny weather in light but mineral-rich and well-drained soil. It is sensitive to cold temperatures and typically do not survive frosts. It is in the Labiatae family.

Properties: Analgesic, antibacterial, anti-depressant, antifungal, antiseptic, antispasmodic, antiviral, carminative, cephalic, diuretic, expectorant, febrifuge, galactagogue, insecticide, mucolytic, nervine, sudorific and tonic.

Chemistry: Phenol (eugenol); Ethers (estragole [methyl chavicol]); Alcohols (linalool; citronellol); Oxides (1,8 cineole); Esters (methyl cinnamate); Monoterpenes (ocimene, linalool) and Ketones.

Main Body Systems: Circulation, digestion, nervous

Physical: Anorexia, bloating, bronchitis, colds, colic, fever, gas, indigestion, headaches, nausea, PMS, nerve pain, restores nervous system communication, scorpion stings, sinus congestion and vein circulation.

Mental: Cognitive strength, depression, fatigue (intellectual and general), melancholy, mental clarity, mental stuckness, nervousness and enhance understanding.

Emotional: Cold-hearted, darkness, depression, feel attacked, hysteria, insomnia (from excessive worry), lack of will, sadness, sensitivity due to "struck a nerve", stress, and sorrow.

Chakra: 1st (root), 3rd (solar plexus), 4th (heart), 7th (crown)

History: Over 200 varieties. In Italy, basil was associated with love. In Greece, it was associated with poverty and misfortune. The Jewish relied on it to bring strength during long periods of fasting. In India it was considered sacred to honor the Hindu Gods. Egypt scattered it on the graves of their departed loved ones.

Personal Experience: I've used sweet basil essential oil in a few different ways. For nerve issues such as nervousness and anxiety, and nerve pain like sciatica and neuropathy. To assist with better digestion and assimilation of nutrients. To clear the mind and provoke positive thinking. And I've had friends tell me it has worked for their phantom limb and paralysis pain and gout.

Contraindications: Noted as a non-irritant.

Bay Laurel (Laurus nobilis)

Scent: Sweet yet dry, floral, warming oil with hints of cinnamon and clove

Note: Middle 7-8, however 1 drop has a high intensity and will go a long way

Extraction Method: Steam distillation

Parts Used: Leaves

Plant Description: It is an evergreen tree or shrub with glossy, dark green leaves, yellow flowers and dark purple to black berries. The tree can reach a height of 40-65-feet and can tolerate strong winds but not maritime (near the sea) exposure. The laurel shrubs can reach 30-feet in height. It prefers dry, well-drained and acidic soil, although it does like to be watered often. It likes a warm, sunlit to semi-shaded area. It is in the Lauraceae family.

Properties: Analgesic, antibacterial, antifungal, antiparasitic, anti-rheumatic, antiseptic, antispasmodic, emmenagogue, febrifuge, rubefacient, stomachic, sudorific, tonic and vulnerary.

Chemistry: Oxides (1,8 cineole); Monoterpinol (linalool, α-terpineol); Monoterpene (pinene, sabinene, myrcene); Esters (terpinyl acetate, geranyl acetate); Phenol (eugenol); Lactones; and Sesquiterpenes.

Main Body Systems: Digestion, nervous, respiratory

Physical: Digestive soother, dizziness, mobility, muscle aches and pains, muscle atrophy (general, phantom limb, para- and quadriplegics), nerve pain, PMS and menopause relief, respiratory support and tonifies liver and kidneys.

Mental: Anxiety, cognitive weakness, concentration, confidence, courage, creativeness, depression, determination, insight, inspiration, increases intuition, insomnia, memory strength, self-esteem and worry.

Emotional: Abandonment, avoid confrontations, egotistical, fear (especially of failure and public speaking), feel defeated, loneliness, passion to conquer a challenge, people pleaser, rejection, self-love, self-worth and victorious.

Chakra: 1st (root), 4th (heart), 6th (third eye)

History: Laurel is most recognized for its use in the Olympic Games as symbol of victory, where laurel wreaths were placed on the heads of winning athletes. Other folklore states that it was said to protect against lightning strikes and negative energies, as well as enhance psychic abilities. It was considered in ancient cultures to be a sacred plant, and a symbol of achievement, wisdom, peace and protection. The leaves are commonly added to soups, casseroles and hot dishes.

Personal Experience: I use this essential oil for nerve pain (physical and emotional), abandonment and separation issues. Its sweetness offers a sense of comfort and feeling wanted.

Contraindications: May cause skin hypersensitivity if used undiluted.

Benzoin *(Stryax benzoin)*

Scent: Deep but light, warm, earth scent with mild sweet, vanilla and mint undertones

Note: Base 8-9

Extraction Method: Solvent Extraction

Parts Used: Resin (resinoid)

Plant Description: Other recognized common names are onycha and Benjamin tree. A large tropical evergreen shrub or tree that can grow 65-100 feet tall. It is a quick-growing tree with deep green, ovate leaves. It has 5-petal white pendulous flowers with several yellow, skinny stamens in the center, and produce drupes. The tree has strong branches and soft bark, from which the resin is extracted. After the tree is injured or cut, a milky resin exudes from the bark. When it becomes an essential oil, it turns into a golden-brown color. It is in the Styracaceae family.

Properties: Analgesic, antibacterial, antidepressant, anti-inflammatory, antiseptic, antiviral, decongestant, expectorant, febrifuge, preservative, stimulant, styptic, vasoconstrictor and vulnerary.

Chemistry: Esters (Coniferyl benzoate, benzoic acid, cynnamyl benzoate); Aldehydes (vanillin); and Alcohols.

Main Body Systems: Respiratory, structural, urinary

Physical: Blood circulation, colds, dandruff, dry and cracked skin, fever, gout, headaches, herpes simplex (fever blisters), hot flashes, indigestion, migraines, nausea, respiratory, scalp nourisher, sinus congestion and urinary support.

Mental: Confidence, depression, exhaustion, focus, imagination, meditation, mental chatter, mental clarity, nervousness, overthinking, PTSD, rejuvenates mind and body, strengthens cognition, stress and worry.

Emotional: Buffers emotional pain, cutting emotions, emotional wounds, grief, inspires connection to accept self, lonely, promotes inner awareness, soothes emotional instability and warms the heart.

Chakra: 1st (root), 3rd (solar plexus), 6th (third eye), 7th (crown)

History: The Egyptians, Greeks and Romans used benzoin often in incense burning concoctions. In the 17th century Great Plague of England, it was combined with frankincense to destroy the "aura" of diseases. It has long been used in cooking, chewing gum, tea and toothpaste for its preservative and therapeutic benefits. It is commonly used in perfumes as a fixative.

Personal Experience: I use this essential oil for dry, cracked and chapped skin issues, as well as to enhance respiratory and urinary functions. Emotionally, it brings a warmth to my heart and lungs, thus promoting love, self-love and grief relief. A deep nourisher.

Contraindications: Non-toxic

Bergamot *(Citrus bergamia; bergaterpene free)*

Scent: Sweet, citrus scent with floral notes

Note: Top

Extraction Method: Steam Distillation

Parts Used: Fruit rind

Plant Description: It is an evergreen tree that can grow up to 30 feet tall. It has smooth, glossy green leaves, white, star-shaped flowers and round shaped fruit. It requires full sun exposure (doesn't do well in the shade) and rich, moist but well-drained soil. It is frost sensitive. Bergamot comes from the bitter orange tree which produces two additional oils – Neroli from the flowers and Petitgrain from the leaves. The name bergamot is said to derive from the Italian city of Bergamo, where bergamot oil was first marketed. Legend holds that Christopher Columbus brought the tree to Italy from the Canary Islands. It is in the Rutaceae family.

Properties: Antibacterial, antidepressant, anti-infectious, antiseptic, antispasmodic, antiviral, astringent, cicatrisant, digestive, febrifuge, insecticide, rubefacient, stomachic and vulnerary.

Chemistry: Monoterpenes (limonene, pinene, myrcene); Furanocoumarins (bergaptene, bergaptole); Monoterpenols (linalool, geraniol); Esters (linalyl acetate, geranyl acetate); Sesquiterpenes (caryophyllene) Aldehydes and Coumarins.

Bergapten-free Bergamot (safe for sun exposure)

Main Body Systems: Immune, nervous, structural

Physical: Acne, addictions, autonomic nervous system (ANS) support, deodorant, digestive aid, fever blisters, fevers, hemorrhoids, libido, mouth sores, oily skin, shingles, sore throat, stop smoking aid, sore throat, urinary issues and vein support.

Mental: Addictions, anxiety, depression, fatigue, mental clarity, mood swings, nervousness, obsessive and compulsive, post-partum, Seasonal Affective Disorder (SAD) and stress.

Emotional: Agitated, anger, bitterness, closed-heartedness, contentment, depression, discouragement, frustration, gloomy, irritability, joy, resentment, shock, speak up for self, timid and trauma.

Chakra: 4th (heart), 5th (throat), 6th (third eye), 7th (crown)

History: Used often n perfumeries and medicine in France since 16th century. Used to flavor Earl Grey Tea and sometimes added to tobacco for flavoring. The British ladies used to sit and drink Earl Grey tea while their husbands were out hunting.

Personal Experience: I use this essential oil to lift mood, combat sugar cravings (along with cinnamon), calm skin irritations, in my homemade deodorant and for viral issues. Emotionally it is great to combat depression, sadness, feeling defeated and uninspired.

 Contraindications: Photosensitive, so avoid direct sunlight 9-12 hours after use on skin. Bergaterpene-free is safer for sun exposure.

Birch *(Betula lenta, alleghaniensis)*

Scent: Sharp, sweet, fresh, minty, camphoraceous with slight green undertones

Note: Middle 6

Extraction Method: Steam Distillation

Parts Used: Bark

Plant Description: Referred to often as a pioneer species, taking root where most would not. It grows at a fast rate, and reach heights of 79 feet. It has a thin trunk with whitish-grey bark that is dark brown when it breaks or flakes off. The yellow and green leaves are tear shaped with serrated edges, and have long braid-like seed stands with a hard texture. It likes dry, well-drained, acidic soil and thrives in the shade to no shade areas. It is a part of the Betulaceae family.

Chemistry: Phenols (methyl salycilate); Carboxylic Acids (salicylic acid); Triterpenes (betula saponins); and Oxides

Main Body Systems: Immune, nervous, structural

Properties: Analgesic, anti-arthritic, antibacterial, antifungal, antigalactagogue, anti-inflammatory, antiseptic, diaphoretic, diuretic, expectorant, febrifuge, insecticide and stimulant.

Physical: Bee stings, bladder and kidney issues, circulation support, digestive upset, edema, enhances elimination, fever, gout, lung ailments, muscle and joint pain and stiffness, nausea, neuralgia, rheumatism, sinus support, stomach aches, toothaches and urinary issues.

Mental: Alertness, awareness, concentration, flexible thinking, focus, headaches, memory, mentally drained, migraines, problem solving and opens up and refreshes the mind.

Emotional: Acceptance of oneself, aggravation, anger, courage, emotional pain, emotional flexibility, fear, feel attacked and invaded, inferiority complex, feel truncated, suffocated by circumstances and trauma.

Chakra: 3rd (solar plexus), 5th (chakra), 6th (third eye)

History: An old English recipe uses the sap, fermented, to make birch beer or vinegar. Ancient cultures used it to tighten and tone skin. Native North American Indians used as a blood purifier, acting to cleanse the body by its emetic and cathartic properties, air purifier around the sick and to flavor medicines. Many cultures say it symbolizes purification, renewal and protection. Today, birch bark is used as a fragrance component in men's perfumes, and more extensively as a flavoring agent in chewing gum, toothpaste and especially in root beer.

Personal Experience: I use this essential oil for a couple different reasons. I like it for muscle stiffness and pain, to keep me alert and focused when studying and driving, to clear my sinuses and to renew my spirit. It also helps with emotional pain, distress, confusion and lethargy.

Contraindications: Contains methyl salicylate, the active ingredient in aspirin. Avoid with blood thinning medications, those who bruise and bleed easily (like the elderly), pregnancy or nursing and with severe liver ailments. May cause skin irritations and burns, especially when used undiluted.

Black Pepper *(Piper nigrum)*

Scent: Spicy, warm, woody with slight bittersweet undertone

Note: Middle 6-7

Extraction Method: Steam Distillation

Part Used: Dried black peppercorns/fruit

Plant Description: It is a perennial vine that grows along a stake, and can reach 18 feet high. It has dark green, oval, heart-shaped leaves, small white flowers and strands of green, red and black berries. It requires hydration but well-drained, rich soil, in hot and humid climates in partial shade. It is frost sensitive and drought tolerant. It is a member of the Piperaceae family.

Properties: Analgesic, antibacterial, antiviral, antiseptic, analgesic, antispasmodic, aphrodisiac, carminative, diaphoretic, diuretic, diaphoretic, febrifuge, rubefacient, stimulant and tonic.

Chemistry: Monoterpenes (piperine, limonene, pinene, sabinene, phellandrene, thujene, camphrene); Sesquiterpenes (caryophyllene, selinene, bisabolene, farnesene); Oxides (caryophyllene oxide); Monoterpinol (linalool); Ketones; Aldehydes; and Furanocoumarins *(http://pubs.acs.org/doi/abs/10.1021/jf60071a008)*.

Main Body Systems: Circulatory (brain and body), nervous, urinary

Physical: Arthritis, blood circulation, bruises, cold and flu, constipation, digestive aid, fibromyalgia, heart health, lymphatic congestion, muscle and joint pain, neuralgia, sciatica, sore throat, toothaches and vein health (capillaries, varicose).

Mental: Alertness, clear thinking, concentration, confidence, depression, focus headaches, gut-brain communication, courage, hesitant, indecision, inspiration, memory, mental fatigue, motivation, sluggishness and worry.

Emotional: Bitterness, emotional endurance to manage challenges, emotionally stuck, frustrated things aren't moving, insecure, irritability, lack of compassion, open up and express feelings, resentment, self-worth and untrusting, weakness.

Chakra: 2nd (sacral), 3rd (solar plexus), 5th (throat), 6th (third eye)

History: Pepper was first described in India's Sanskrit literature 3,000 years ago, and primarily used for liver and urinary disorders. Romans, Germans and English used it in place of currency to pay their taxes, bills and barter. For a long time, it was the most important commodity in world trade. It is one of the most widely used spices in culinary dishes to add flavor, spice and stimulate digestion. Used in the Middle Ages in Europe to season and preserve meat and mask rancid food odors. Studies show it enhances the absorption of curcumin, vitamin B, beta carotene and selenium *(http://www.ncbi.nlm.nih.gov/pubmed/25618800)*.

Personal Experience: I use this essential oil to stimulate circulation, combat indigestion, warm extremities and for vein support. Emotionally it helps to decongest stuck, numb emotions, freeing the mind of insecurity, and instilling confidence and pride.

✶ **Contraindications**: May cause skin irritations if not in a carrier. ✶

✓Blue Cypress (*Callitris intratropica*)

Scent: Woody, warm, earthy with slight sweet and balsamic undertones

Note: Middle-Base 6-7

Extraction Method: Steam Distillation

Parts Used: Wood and/or needles

Plant Description: Also known as Northern Australian cypress pine, is a tall, aromatic evergreen tree, reaching heights of 75 feet. It has blue-green leaves that have a feather-like bristle appearance, along strong branches that fan to the sides forming a semi-pyramidal shape. It has small, tulip-looking seed-containing cones. The wood is strong and a natural insecticide. It prefers to be grown in sandy, well-drained soils in the warm, rainy weather, but is tolerant of most climates. It is in the Cupressaceae family.

Chemistry: Sesquiterpenols (guaiol, eudesmol, bulnesol); and Sesquiterpenes (elemene, selinene, guaiazulene).

Main Body Systems: Circulatory, muscular-skeletal, nervous

Properties: Analgesic, antibacterial, anti-inflammatory, antiparasitic, antispasmodic, antiviral, carminative, emmenagogue, insecticide, sedative and vulnerary.

Physical: Acne, bone strength, cold sores, diarrhea, digestive upset, joint pain and swelling, hemorrhoids, intestinal spasms, parasites, PMS, rheumatoid arthritis, shingles, skin irritations, sprains, urinary support and wet coughs.

Mental: Anxiety, indecisive, determination, focus, insomnia, moving forward in a direction, nervousness, perfectionist, speaking articulately and wisdom.

Emotional: Encouragement, emotional stabilizer, emotional wounds, fear of failure, feel "burned" by someone, grounding, hopeful, protection, reassuring, security, stable, strength, stress and survival.

Chakra: 4th (heart), 5th (throat), 6th (third eye)

History: Distilled for the first time in 1996, it is a newer essential oil. Indigenous to Australia and the Tiwi tribe, they used it to make spear shafts, musical instruments and soap. It has been used for firewood, since it burns good and keeps the mosquitoes away. It was used medicinally for its antispasmodic, analgesic and pest control.

Personal Experience: I use this essential oil for acne, muscle fatigue, mental exhaustion and anxiety. It makes me feel grounded, connected and at peace with my decisions.

Contraindications: Avoid during pregnancy. Not recommended for internal use. Mild skin irritant.

Blue Tansy – see *Tanacetum annuum*

Cajuput *(Melaleuca cajeputi)*

Scent: Strong, opening, medicinal, camphoraceous with slight fruit undertones.

Note: Middle but one drop in a blend goes a long way.

Extraction Method: Steam Distillation

Parts Used: Leaves and twigs

Plant Description: It is either a small or large evergreen tree, with heights up to 45-120 feet. The trunk is usually long, sometimes crooked with soft, thick, spongy and whitish-colored bark. The branches droop similar to the weeping willow with lanceolate leaves that are very aromatic. It produces small clusters of hair-like white flowers that have no scent. It prefers to be grown in dry, well-drained, acidic soils in the direct sunlight. It does not do well in the shade. It is in the Myrtaceae family.

Chemistry: Oxides (1,8 cineole); Monoterpenes (limonene, pinene, cymene); Monoterpenols (terpineol); Sesquiterpenes (caryophyllene); Sesquiterpinols; Aldehydes; and Esters.

Main Body Systems: Immune, respiratory, structural

Properties: Analgesic, antibacterial, antifungal, antiparasitic, antiseptic, antispasmodic, diaphoretic, expectorant, insecticide and stimulant (immune).

Physical: Colds, earaches, headaches and migraines, immunity, muscles aches and pains, neuralgia, respiratory concerns and congestion, rheumatism, sinus issues and toothaches.

Mental: Balances the mind body connection, clears the mind, concentration, focus, enhancing listening skills, indecisive, mental chatter and scattered and wandering thoughts.

Emotional: Anger, agitation, emotional sluggishness, fear of others invading their space, feeling suffocated with no room to breathe, feeling suppressed, irritability, tragedy and trauma support and excessive worry.

Chakra: 3rd (solar plexus), 4th (heart), 5th (throat)

History: Closely related to niaouli and tea tree, but different. Cajeput has been referred to as the paperbark tree, or swamp tea tree. In the 1700's and 1800's, it was commonly used for developing industry tools and warfare since the wood is soft and flexible. The wood also served as an insecticide. It is used in analgesic ointments in Traditional Chinese Medicine. Indonesia and Vietnam considered it to be a tree of protection. It is believed that inhaling the scent can enhance willpower and innate focus.

Personal Experience: I use this essential oil to open respiratory channels, promote alertness and mental focus, combat congestion, muscle soreness and pain and I diffuse it to boost immunity.

Contraindications: This can be a very irritating oil to the skin and internal organs. Do not use internally as it can be toxic to the nervous system, liver (especially when in distress) and the gastro-intestinal tract or biliary ducts. Avoid during pregnancy.

Camphor, White (*Cinnamomum camphora*)

Scent: Strong, penetrating, refreshing scent with sweet undertones

Note: Middle

Extraction Method: Steam Distillation

Parts Used: Wood, roots, branches

Plant Description: It is a fire-resistant, evergreen tree that is native to Asia. It can grow up to 50-150 feet and has a wide trunk. It has smooth braches with alternating leaves, that when crushed, disperse its camphor scent. It has tiny, cream-colored flowers that produce many round, pea-sized purple-black berries. The camphor tree can grow in full sun or partial shade, with fertile, sandy, alkaline soil. It grows poorly in wet soils. Mature trees can be drought tolerant as well as survive freezes. Their root systems can multiply quickly especially as they get older, which sometimes can smother surrounding areas. It is a member of the Lauraceae family. This tree produces two essential oils, camphor from the wood and ho leaf from the leaves.

Properties: Analgesic, antigalactagogue, anti-inflammatory, anti-rheumatic, aphrodisiac, carminative, diaphoretic, expectorant, febrifuge, stimulant and vulnerary.

Chemistry: Ketones (fenchone, thujone, piperitone); Oxides (1,8 cineole); Monoterpinol (borneol); Diterpenes (camphorene); Monoterpenes (pinene, camphene, limonene); and Phenols (safrole).

Main Body Systems: Circulatory, respiratory, structural

Physical: Acne, bronchitis, circulation, cold sores, fever, headaches, muscle and joint pain, neuralgia, respiratory issues, sinusitis, skin diseases, stamina and toothaches.

Mental: Alertness, coma, clarity, concentration, depression, determination, domineering, fainting or light-headed, focus, mental fatigue, nervousness and traumatic brain injuries.

Emotional: Balances emotions, cold hearted, grounding, opening (up heart, mind, possibilities and crown chakra), refreshing, rejuvenating to the mind, body and spirit, suffocated and weepiness.

Chakra: 6th (third eye), 7th (crown)

History: Most popular for its medicinal and analgesic use in Asia. The Chinese also used the wood to build ships and temples due to its durability and aromatic quality. In Persia they used it to protect against the plague. Camphor has been historically used as an insecticide, especially for moths, in ceremonies and rituals, and in embalming agents. See Ho Leaf essential oil for explanation of the botanical name.

Personal Experience: I use this essential oil to open up my sinuses, enhance mental clarity and stamina, alleviate sore muscles and disinfect acne (in a carrier). Emotionally it can help you open up with freedom from suppression.

 Contraindications: Avoid during pregnancy, with epilepsy and asthmatics.

Cardamom *(Elettaria cardamomum)*

Scent: Spicy with sweet, pungent, vegetative, camphoraceous notes

Note: Middle 5-6

Extraction Method: Steam Distillation

Parts Used: Fruit and/or seeds

Plant Description: It is an aromatic perennial shrub that can grow up to 6-12 feet high. It has strong shoots or long stems with long semi-floppy leaves. At the base, strong skinny, stick-like stems grow that produce pods or fruits that encase the cardamom seeds as well as white-purplish flowers. It requires constant moisture and warm temperatures with partial shade. It is a member of the Zingiberaceae family.

Properties: Analgesic, anti-inflammatory, antibacterial, antispasmodic, aphrodisiac, carminative, diaphoretic, digestive, diuretic, expectorant, nutritive, stomachic and stimulant.

Chemistry: Esters (terpinyl acetate, linalyl acetate); Oxides (1,8 cineole); Alcohols (linalool terpineol, terpin-4-ol); Monoterpenes (limonene, sabinene, myrcene); and Sesquiterpenes (trans-nerolidol).

Main Body Systems: Digestion, respiratory, urinary

Physical: Acid reflux, cough, digestive discomfort, GI issues, fever, intestinal spasms, liver issues, nausea, over-exertion, PMS, respiratory concerns, urinary issues and tooth and gum issues.

Mental: Concentration, confusion, depression, dizziness, exhaustion, headache, memory recall, mental fatigue, nervous exhaustion, overthinking and worry.

Emotional: Anxiety, cold-heart, confidence, contentment, emotionally drained, fear, inspiration, lifts mood, restores vital chi and inner passion, sadness, warms the heart and calms weepiness.

Chakra: 1st (root), 2nd (sacral), 3rd (solar plexus), 4th (heart)

History: In India, it was and still is used as a culinary spice with medicinal benefits. It is most popular today in chai tea. It has been called the "queen of spices". The ancient Greeks and Romans used it in food dishes, medicine and perfumes. Traditional Chinese Medicine uses it for stomach and digestive problems. Egyptians chewed cardamom to sweeten their breath and whiten their teeth.

Personal Experience: I use this essential oil for digestive upset, silent reflux, chronic cough, weakened chi and dry ailments. Emotionally, it warm my heart, makes me feel nourished and loved.

Contraindications: Non-irritating.

Carrot Seed *(Daucus carota)*

Scent: Woody, earthy scent with hints of sweet and fresh undertones

Note: Middle 5-6

Extraction Method: Steam distillation

Parts Used: Seeds

Plant Description: It is a biennial herb with a tough, taproot. The stalks grow above ground and can reach three feet tall. The carrot itself grows beneath the soil and takes two years to grow to fruition. Its stems and leaves are covered with coarse hairs. It does not produce its clusters of tiny white flowers until its second year, and then it dies. It thrives best in loose, rich, well-drained soil grown in full sun with lots of moisture. It is a member of the Umbelliferae family.

Chemistry: Monoterpenols (carotol, daucol, linalool); Monoterpenes (pinene, sabinene, limonene); Sesquiterpenes (bisabolene, caryophyllene); Oxides (caryophyllene oxide); Esters (geranyl acetate); Tetraterpenes; and Phenols.

Main Body Systems: Hepatic, lymphatic, structural

Properties: Antibacterial, antioxidant, antiviral, antifungal, analgesic, anti-inflammatory, diuretic, hepatic, galactagogue, trophorestorative, vulnerary and vasodilative.

Physical: Eyesight, heart palpitations, hepatitis, kidney and liver support, left-sided issues, lymph stagnation and drainage, skin issues (dry, sensitive, mature, roseacea, scars, pigmentation) and improves skin collagen and elasticity.

Mental: Anxiety, clear physic blocks and clutter, confused and disconnected, enhance inner vision, exhaustion, mental chatter, mental clarity, stamina and nervousness.

Emotional: Challenges with females, courage, emotional stuckness due to pain, fear, feel isolated and alone, insecurity, promote joy, mother nurturing, nourish emotional balance and unprotected.

Chakra: 1st (root), 3rd (solar plexus), 5th (throat), 6th (third eye)

History: Its common name is "Queen Anne's lace." Because it has been noted to contain high amounts of vitamins and minerals (i.e. carotene), it has been a popular choice to nourish the immune, nervous and structural systems, especially for skin concerns such as sun-damaged skin, discolorations and irritations. The Egyptians, Greeks and Romans used often for medicinal purposes and as an aphrodisiac. In 13th Century Europe it was used for animal bites and as an antiviral.

Personal Experience: I use this essential oil in many of my skin care products such as my cleanser and moisturizer for discoloration and maturing skin. I've also used it during times of fatigue, exhaustion and stress to restore my inner energy, feel nourished and nurtured as well self-love.

Contraindications: Non-irritating.

Cassia *(Cinnamomum cassia)*

Scent: Spicy, hot, sharp scent with sweet, pungent, wood undertones

Note: Middle 6-7

Extraction Method: Steam distillation

Parts used: Bark, leaves, twigs

Plant Description: Also referred to as Chinese cinnamon. It is an evergreen tree with slender trunks that can grow to heights of 30-50 feet. The bark is thick and darker in color than cinnamon. The bark is harvested by peeling it back and letting it dry in the sun. The leaves are green (red when young), fern-like shape that grow outward forming a canopy with slick, firm yellow flowers grown in clusters that emit its rich, spicy scent. It needs lots of rain, heat and sheltered areas with consistent temperatures. It prefers nutrient-rich, well-drained but dry soil. The bark is a cinnamon brown color. It is a member of the Lauraceae family.

Chemistry: Aldehydes (transcinnamaldehyde, methoxycinnam-aldehyde); Coumarins; Phenols (eugenol); Esters (cinnamyl acetate, benzyl acetate); Monoterpenols and Carboxylic Acids.

Main Body Systems: Circulatory, intestinal, immune

Properties: Analgesic, antibacterial, anti-inflammatory, antiparasitic, antiseptic, antispasmodic, antiviral, aphrodisiac, astringent, nervine, stimulant and vermifuge.

Physical: Appetite stimulant, colds and flu, cold extremities, diabetes, digestive aid, gastrointestinal issues, immune support, low blood pressure, parasites, PMS, respiratory concerns, sore muscles and toothache.

Mental: Alert, anxiety, confusion, creativity, depression, exhaustion, indecision, joy, mental health imbalances, mood swings, nervous, panic, resentment, sleepiness and stress.

Emotional: Abandonment, bitterness, deep emotional pain, emotional strength, emotionally cold, fear, grief, guilt, lonely, security, self-esteem, suppression and warms a weak heart.

Chakra: 2nd (sacral), 3rd (solar plexus), 5th (throat)

History: One of the oldest spices known to man. It is notes several times in the bible and used in many ancient cultures for its medicinal benefits such as digestion, immune and toothaches. It is also common in many food dishes for its gastrointestinal support as well as mouthwashes and toothpastes for its anti-infectious properties. It is also less expensive than cinnamon.

Personal Experience: I use this essential oil for a room disinfectant, to bring me warmth when I am chilly, stimulate circulation, ignite my fire to be motivated and warms my heart.

Contraindications: Avoid if taking blood thinners as it may inhibit blood clotting (more than Cinnamomum zylancium). Do not use internally as it maybe irritating the membranes. Do not use undiluted as it is a known skin irritant. Minimize use with high blood pressure. Avoid if pregnant as it contains some abortifacient properties.

Catnip (Nepeta cataria)

Scent: Herbaceous with sweet, citronella-mint like undertones

Note: Middle 5-6

Extraction Method: Steam Distillation

Parts Used: Leaves and/or flowers

Plant Description: It is an herbal plant that can grow up to 3 feet high. It has heart-shaped green leaves with serrated edges, and when crushed it emits a stronger odor. It produces tiny white-purplish flowers in cone-shaped stems. It prefers dry climates, thus it is drought tolerant, in full sunlight with minimal shade and watering. It thrives in well-drained, sandy, alkaline soil. It is a member of the Labiatae family.

Properties: Analgesic, antibacterial, anti-inflammatory, antispasmodic, antiviral, astringent, carminative, digestive, diuretic, emmenagogue, expectorant, insecticide, stimulant and tonic.

Chemistry: Monoterpenols (citronellol, geraniol, nerol); Lactone (nepetalactone); Aldehydes (geranial, neral); Sesquiterpenes (caryophyllene, humulene); Monoterpenes (myrcene); and Phenols.

Main Body Systems: Digestive, immune, respiratory

Physical: Colic, coughs (dry) digestive upset, intestinal spasms, immune support, joint swelling, nausea, PMS, respiratory support and urinary issues.

Mental: Anxiety, behavioral issues, concentration, courage, creativity, depression, headache, insomnia, mental fatigue, nervous, nightmares and shock.

Emotional: Agitation, anger, compulsive, despair, emotional exhaustion, grief, inspires having fun without being burdened by responsibilities, obsessive, sorrow and vulnerability.

Chakra: 1st (root), 2nd (sacral), 3rd (solar plexus), 5th (throat), 7th (crown)

History: Most popular for its effect on cats when they rub up against it and release its euphoric scent. It also is a popular rat, mice, ants, fleas, insect and beetle repellent. Some scientists have found that a larger percentage of mosquitoes are repelled by catnip extract versus DEET. The Greeks and Romans used medicinally for immunity. In France, it is commonly used as a culinary spice, as it enhances digestion. Europe uses is as a relaxant, headache and digestive aid, even with children.

Personal Experience: I use this essential oil in my insect and flea repellent, in addition to calming digestive upset, boosting immune function and inspiring creative, positive thinking.

Contraindications: Avoid during pregnancy. Not for ingestion. May cause skin sensitivity.

Cedars

There are four closely related species of true cedars today - *Cedrus atlantica* (Atlas cedar), *Cedrus deodara* (Himalayan cedar), *Cedrus libani* (Lebanon cedar, endangered) and *Cedrus brevifolia* (native to Cyprus). I will discuss the first two, Atlas and Himalayan Cedars since these are more widely used in aromatherapy. You will notice many similarities, but there are a few differences especially when it comes to chemistry, thus diversity in properties and benefits.

Atlas *(Cedrus atlantica)*

Scent: Woody, warm, hearty earth scent with sweet balsamic undertones

Note: Middle to Upper Base 7-8

Extraction Method: Steam Distillation

Parts Used: Wood

Plant Description: It is a hardy, pyramid-shaped, furry-looking evergreen that can live for centuries. It does like space around it and can grow up to 60 feet high. The silver-blue-ish leaves are comprised of small bristles that are firm, however the branches are semi-flexible and flow in the wind. It produces green-brownish colored, oblong cones that have a tight, woven enclosed exterior. The wood is reddish-brown. It grows best in full sunlight, prefers moist, acidic and well-drained soil. Older trees can tolerate drought (hot and dry) and milder winds. Native to Morocco and Atlas Mountains. It is a member of the Pinaceae family.

Properties: Antiviral, antibacterial, antiseptic, astringent, carminative, cephalic, diuretic, antispasmodic, emmenagogue, expectorant, febrifuge, insecticide, mucolytic and sedative.

Chemistry: Sesquiterpenes (himachalene, cadinene); Sesquiterpenols (alantol, caryophellenol, cubenol, cedrol); and Sesquiterpenones (alantone).

Main Body Systems: Cephalic, circulation, respiration, urinary

Physical: Acne, adrenal exhaustion, arthritis, bronchitis, constipation, cystitis, dandruff, eczema and psoriasis, joint pain, kidney and urinary issues, lower back pain, nervousness, oily skin, physical strength and skin irritations.

Mental: Anxiety, balances mental thoughts, concentration, depression, focus, learning abilities, melancholy, mental performance and strength, nervous tension (especially due to endocrine system imbalances) and spiritually harmonizing.

Emotional: Anger, courage, desire, emotional strength, fear, grounding, insecurity, paranoia, protects against "people parasites", stamina to withstand heavy burden, warms the heart and facilitates willpower.

Chakra: 1st (root), 2nd (sacral) and 3rd (solar plexus), 6th (third eye), 7th (crown)

History: The wood is highly prized and most notable for its wood strength and natural insect deterrent aroma. It was and still is commonly used to build wooden structures such as furniture, fences and treehouses. In ancient times, used to construct temples, palaces and ship masts. Ancient Egyptians used it in the embalming process and in perfumes. The Bible references cedar trees as a symbol of fertility and abundance.

Personal Experience: I love this essential oil for mental focus and concentration especially when there is adrenal fatigue and mineral deficiencies. It instills a sense of strength in the neck (at the occiput), all the way down the spine to our tailbone. I've seen children with learning and cognitive issues behave with more discipline, focus and alertness, mental performance (in autism).

Contraindications: Non-irritating.

Himalayan *(Cedrus deodorata)*

Scent: Deep woodsy and earthy scent with hints of a slightly sweet and fresh camphor

Note: Middle to Upper base, 7-8

Extraction Method: Steam Distillation

Parts Used: Wood

Plant Description: Similar to *Cedrus atlantica*, it is a shaggy, pyramid-shaped evergreen that can grow on average up to 70 feet in height, and sometimes to a height if 250 feet in the Himalayas. It has silver-blue-ish leaves that are comprised of stiff small bristles located on semi-flexible but durable branches. It produces green-brownish colored, oblong cones, larger than that of the *Cedrus atlantica*, and have tight, woven enclosed exterior. The wood is reddish-brown. It grows best in full sunlight, prefers moist, acidic and well-drained soil. It is drought tolerant, can withstand mild winds but more sensitive to pollution. Native to the Himalayas and a member of the Pinaceae family.

Properties: Antiviral, antibacterial, antiseptic, astringent, carminative, diaphoretic, diuretic, antispasmodic, emmenagogue, expectorant, insecticide and sedative.

Chemistry: Sesquiterpenes (cadinene, himachalene); Sesquiterpenols (alantol, caryophellenol, cedrol); Sesquiterpenones (alantone); Monoterpenes (limonene); Monoterpenols (linalool, terpineol); and Ethers (anethole).

Main Body Systems: Glandular, muscular-skeletal and respiratory

Physical: Acne, arthritis, bruising, carminative, coughs, cystitis, dandruff, digestive upset, eczema and psoriasis, fevers, joint pain, lower back pain, kidney/adrenal exhaustion, oily skin, physical strength, skin irritations, snake bites and urinary tract issues.

Mental: Anxiety, concentration, connect to inner self, depression, grounding, insomnia, nervousness, mental performance (especially when there are deficiencies) and strength, opens up higher thinking, rejuvenates soul and sadness.

Emotional: Anger, courage, defend against negativity, desire, emotional strength, enhances spirituality stability, fear, grounding, insecurity, paranoia, stamina to withstand heavy burden and willpower.

Chakra: 1st (root), 2nd (sacral) and 3rd (solar plexus), 6th (third eye), 7th (crown)

History: Hindu cultures consider this to be a divine tree. The wood is highly durable, a natural insecticide and rot-resistant, thus making it a popular wood for building structures, buildings, temples, barracks, bridges, canals and boats. It has been used in Ayurveda medicines especially for pulmonary concerns. It is a common ingredient in perfumes, soaps and cleaning solutions. It has been called "the most graceful Cedar" by tree expert and author, Michael Dirr.

Personal Experience: I use this essential oil for mental, emotional and spiritual grounding, to make me "stand tall" and open myself up to the bigger picture. I also like it to help enhance my breathing, calm cough, balance my nerves and strengthen my cognitive functions.

Contraindications: Non-irritating.

Celery Seed *(Apium graveolens)*

Scent: Warm, earthy, bourbon-like scent with hints of acrid pepper notes

Note: Middle 5

Extraction Method: Steam Distillation

Parts Used: Wood

Plant Description: It is a biennial herbal plant that grows up to 3 feet high. It has a tall, rigid stock with a bulbous rootstock. The leaves are parsley-like that flourish at the top ends and produce tiny white or yellow, clusters of flowers that produce seeds. It grows best in damp, acid soils in cool climates that are semi-shaded to sunny. It is a member of the Umbelliferae family.

Properties: Abortifacient, antiviral, antibacterial, anti-inflammatory, antispasmodic, aphrodisiac, carminative, diaphoretic, diuretic, emmenagogue, galactagogue, insecticide, nervine and tonic.

Chemistry: Monoterpene (limonene, ocimene, terpinene); Esters (carvyl acetate); Lactones (butylphthalide, sedanolides); Sesquiterpenes (selinene); Ketones (carvone); Carboxylic Acids (sedanolic acid); and Monoterpinols.

Main Body Systems: Digestive, glandular, urinary

Physical: Adrenal support, chilblains, circulation, cystitis, edema, gout, indigestion, kidney purifier, laryngitis, liver strengthening, lowers blood pressure, lymphatic congestion, parasites, rheumatism, thyroid support, urinary issues and uterine tonic.

Mental: Anxiety, defensive, exhaustion, fidgety, headaches, insomnia, mental congestion and fatigue, nervousness, overloaded, panic, perfectionist and self-esteem.

Emotional: Anger, despair, emotionally sluggish, encourage gentleness, fear (in general and of death), feel bogged down and swampy, grief, shyness, strength and flexibility, stimulate passion and desire and worthiness.

Chakra: 3rd (solar plexus), 4th (heart); 5th (throat)

History: It was a symbol of grief and death for both the Egyptians and Romans, as they made garlands and wreaths for funerals. The Greeks and Romans used often as a food spice for digestion. They also used it to make wine served as an award at athletic games as well as a hangover remedy. Ayurveda medicine used it to treat colds, flu, edema, poor digestion and arthritis. Studies today are showing benefits in helping lower blood pressure and cholesterol.

Personal Experience: I use this essential oil for urinary and kidney support, swelling of the ankles and joints, bloating, edema and as a digestive aid. I also use it to enhance detoxification of the kidney, lymph, liver and gall bladder. Emotionally it clears out the mental congestions, helping me to think clearly and confidently. It warms the heart and helps me move through stuckness.

Contraindications: Avoid during pregnancy as it is a uterine tonic. May have blood thinning effect. Photosensitive.

Chamomiles

German Chamomile *(Matricaria recutita)*

Scent: Earthy, sweet with hint of green apple scent

Note: Middle 6

Extraction Method: Steam distillation

Parts Used: Flower tops

Plant Description: A perennial evergreen plant that grows up to 3 feet in height, taller than Roman chamomile. The feather-like green leaves are coarser then Roman chamomile with white flowers and a hollow coned yellow center. It prefers dry (but watered daily), well-drained, alkaline soil in a semi-shaded, but not full shade area in warmer climates. It is a member of the Compositae family. The essential oil produced is blue in color.

Chemistry: Oxides (bisabolol oxide, bisabolone, 1,8 cineole); Sesquiterpenes (farnesene, chamazulene, cadinene, muurolene); Sesquiterpenols (bisabolol, farnesol); Ethers (spiro ether); Monoterpenes; and Esters.

Main Body Systems: Digestion, glandular, nervous, urinary

Properties: Analgesic, antibacterial, antidepressant, antifungal, anti-inflammatory, antispasmodic, carminative, cholagogue, cicatrisant, nervine, sedative, stomachic and vulnerary.

Physical: Digestive aid, headaches, hemorrhoids, hiatal hernia, intestinal upset and spasms, motion sickness, muscles aches, pains and spasms, PMS, skin issues, urinary tract and renal issues.

Mental: Anxiety, chaos, insomnia, irritability, mental chatter and stress, neuralgia, nervous irritability, overstimulation, panic attacks, patience, perfectionist, restless and worry excessively.

Emotional: Abandonment, anger, caretaker (and being taken care of), emotional abuse, fear, grief, guilt, harmony, hot/short tempers ("road rage"), jealousy, oversensitive, past hurts, peace, and self-worth.

Chakra: 1st (root), 3rd (solar plexus), 4th (heart), 5th (throat), 7th (crown)

History: Egyptians used for fever with chills that plagued their civilization. Greeks used for baths, headaches and urinary and liver disorders. Common in herbal teas and to flavor beers. In the Middle Ages, it was purposely planted in garden walkways as it emits its aroma when walked up.

Personal Experience: I use this essential oil to nourish my adrenals and glandular systems, as well as enhance vital energy without overstimulation. It makes me feel calm, cool and collected but focused and motivated. I have found it to help when I have inflammation, bruising, swelling, digestive upset, mental chatter and excessive worry.

Contraindications: Avoid if you have ragweed allergies. Photosensitive.

✓ Roman Chamomile *(Anthemis nobilis, Matricaria recutita, Chamaemelum nobile)*

Scent: Earthy, sweet with hint of green apple scent

Note: Middle 5-6

Extraction Method: Steam distillation

Parts Used: Flower tops

Plant Description: A perennial evergreen plant that grows low to the ground, reaching maximum heights of only 12 inches. The feather-like green leaves are semi-soft with daisy-like white flower petals and a golden yellow solid, conical center. It prefers dry (but watered daily), well-drained, alkaline soil, but does okay in most pH soils. It likes a shaded to semi-shaded area, but not full shade, in warm climates. It is drought tolerant as long it's not directly in the sunlight. It is a member of the Compositae family.

Chemistry: Esters (isobutyl angelate, isoamyl methacylate, amyl butyrate, allyl angelate); Monoterpenes (pinene, terpinene, sabinene, limonene); Ketones (pinocarvone); Sesquiterpenes (caryophyllene, chamazulene); Sesquiterpenols (farnesol, nerolidol); Monoterpenols; and Carboxylic Acids.

Main Body Systems: Digestion, glandular, nervous

Properties: Analgesic, antibacterial, antidepressant, antifungal, anti-inflammatory (more than German chamomile), antispasmodic, carminative, febrifuge, nervine, sedative and vulnerary.

Physical: Constipation, digestive aid, diverticulitis, hiatal hernia, intestinal upset and spasms, motion and morning sickness, muscles aches, pains and spasms, peptic ulcers, PMS, urinary tract and renal issues.

Mental: Addictions, antsy, anxiety, communication, concentration, depression, insomnia, loss of control, mental chatter, mental stress and tension, nervous irritability, overstimulation, panic attacks, perfectionist, restlessness, workaholic and worry excessively.

Emotional: Abandonment, caretaker (and being taken care of), compassionate, emotional abuse, fear, grief, guilt, hot/short tempers ("road rage"), individuality, jealousy, loneliness, need nurturing, oversensitive, past hurts, patience, self-worth and spiritual connection.

Chakra: 3rd (solar plexus), 4th (heart), 5th (throat)

History: Egyptians used to anoint their god's and dedicated it to the sun and moon. It was commonly used in perfumes, nervous system medicines and body and hair care. It was planted in many gardens and seemed to do better when walked upon, as it released its aromatic scent. The Middle Ages used it was used as a hop replacement in beers. Most common today in herbal teas and food dishes. It has been often noted gentle enough for children, elderly, pets and those with hypersensitivity.

Personal Experience: I use this essential oil to calm intestinal upset, especially if my IBS and Crohn's flares up, general inflammation like swelling, pain and bruising and to calm my nervous system. Emotionally it has helped me feel nurtured, nourished, loved (self-love), taken care of, appreciated and needed. In reverse, it is for those that need to give those qualities as well. I also add it to my shampoo to enhance golden highlights.

Contraindications: Avoid of you have ragweed allergies.

Cilantro *(Coriandrum sativum)*

Scent: Fresh, green, clean herb-like with earthy, pungent undertones

Note: Middle 5

Extraction Method: Steam distillation

Parts used: Leaves

Plant Description: It is an annual herbal plant that can grow up to 3 feet tall. It has a tall, slender stalk with dark, rich green, feathery leaflets (cilantro). It produces tiny white to pink flowers that turn into small, ribbed, brownish-yellow seeds (coriander) that have a strong odor (becomes better when it is dried). It prefers dry, well-drained, alkaline soil in shaded to semi-shaded areas. It is a member of the Umbelliferae family. This plant also produces coriander which is distilled from the seeds.

Chemistry: Monoterpenols (linalool, coriandrol, geraniol); Monoterpenes (pinene, terpinene, limonene, cymene); Esters (geranyl acetate, linalyl acetate); Ketones (camphor); and Coumarins.

Main Body Systems: Digestive, hepatic, urinary

Properties: Antibacterial, antifungal, anti-halitosis, antispasmodic, antiviral, aphrodisiac carminative, depurative, expectorant, febrifuge, stimulant and stomachic.

Physical: Arthritis, colds, digestive aid, gastrointestinal spasms, liver and lymphatic detoxification, nausea, neuralgia, PMS, rheumatism, urinary support.

Mental: Depression, confusion, dizziness, fatigue, headache, insomnia, learning ability, memory recall with clarity, motivation, nervous, respiratory and stress.

Emotional: Anger, bitterness, disconnectedness, emotional instability, fear (in general and of aging), hopeful, insecure, irritability, joy, laughter, pessimism, refreshed, rejuvenated, self-confidence, shock, undernourished and worry.

Chakra: 1st (root), 2nd (sacral), 4th (heart), 5th (throat), 6th (third eye)

History: The Egyptians believed it to possess the secret to happiness and were used at funerals in the Egyptian tombs. Greek and Romans used it as a medicine to preserve foods, stimulate digestion and calm nerves. Coriander is also employed extensively as a flavoring for gin, and other alcoholic liquors.

Personal Experience: I use this essential oil to enhance kidney and liver detoxification, especially of heavy metals. It also helps balance blood sugar and stimulate digestion. Emotionally, I find it refreshing, rejuvenating and refueling.

Contraindications: Use sparingly with chronic asthma. Can have narcotic effect in high amounts.

Cinnamon *(Cinnamomum zylancium; verum)*

Scent: Spicy, hot, sweet, sharp, clove-like scent

Note: Middle

Extraction Method: Steam distillation

Parts used: Leaf and/or bark

Plant Description: Also referred to as Ceylon Cinnamon. It is an evergreen tree that can grow to heights of 40 feet. It ovate leaves are glossy and red, but as the tree matures, the leaves turn green. It produces blue acorn looking berries. The trunks are slender and have rough bark that flakes off. The bark is harvested by peeling it back, exposing the inner layers, and letting it dry in the sun. It needs lots of rain, heat and sheltered areas with consistent temperatures. It prefers nutrient-rich, well-drained but dry soil. The bark is a reddish-brown color, lighter than cassia. It is a member of the Lauraceae family.

Chemistry: Aldehydes (cinnamaldehyde); Phenols (eugenol, phenol); Monoterpenols (linalool, cinnamic alcohol); Sesquiterpenes (caryophyllene); Esters (benzyl benzoate, eugenol acetate); Carboxylic Acids; and Coumarins.

Main Body Systems: Circulatory, intestinal, immune

Properties: Analgesic, antibacterial, antidiarrheal, antiparasitic, antiseptic, antispasmodic, antiviral, aphrodisiac, astringent, carminative, emmenagogue, stimulant, stomachic and vermifuge.

Physical: Airborne virus, blood sugar imbalance, candida, colds and flu, cold extremities, digestive aid, gastrointestinal issues, immune support, low blood pressure, parasites, PMS, respiratory concerns, silent reflux, sore muscles and toothaches.

Mental: Alertness, anxiety, bitterness, combats sleepiness, confusion, creativity, depression, exhaustion, indecision, joy, mental fatigue, mood swings, nervous, resentment and stress.

Emotional: Abandonment, bereavement, emotional strength, emotionally cold, fear, feel suppressed and not able to reach your full potential, grief, guilt, isolation, lonely, panic, safety, security and warms the heart.

Chakra: 2nd (sacral), 3rd (solar plexus), 5th (throat), 6th (third eye)

History: One of the oldest spices known to man and aphrodisiac. Egyptians used it for embalming. Traditional Chinese Medicine used for many medicinal purposes. It has been noted to disperse unwanted smells and prevent the spread of infection. In Feng Shui, it is said to be the desired scent when trying to sell home as it promotes a warming and inviting feeling. It is also common in many food dishes for its gastrointestinal support.

Personal Experience: I use this essential oil often as a room and hand sanitizer, to lift my mood and energy, promote feelings of comfort, in a bath salt or massage oil for sore muscles and chest congestion, to warm the heart and extremities.

Contraindications: Avoid if taking blood thinners as it may inhibit blood clotting. Do not use internally as it maybe irritating the membranes. Do not use undiluted as it is a known skin irritant. Minimize use with high blood pressure.

high BP

Cistus (*Cistus ladanifer, labdanum*)

Scent: Earthy, camphoraceous with hints of fresh herby wood unfolding

Note: Middle 5-6

Extraction Method: Steam Distillation

Parts Used: Resins, bark, leaf and/or flowers

Plant Description: Also known as rock rose. A fast-growing evergreen shrub that can grow to a height of 8 feet tall. The green, ovate leaves have fine hairs that exude a sticky resin, especially when warm. It produces white flowers in the shape of an upside-down umbrella with small purple ovals near the middle of the yellow, attached center. It likes sunny, dry climates and prefers sandy, acid and well-drained soil. It does not transplant well once it has matured. It is drought and wind tolerant and can adapt to wildfires. It is a member of the Cistaceae family.

Chemistry: Monoterpenes (pinene, camphene, cadinene, limonene); Monoterpenols (terpineol, pinocarveol, borneol); Esters (bornyl acetate, methyl benzoate, linalyl acetate); Ketones (cyclohexanone, fenchone); Aldehydes (benzylaldehyde); Diterpenols (labdanenol); and Carboxylic Acids.

Main Body Systems: Immune, nervous, structural

Properties: Antibacterial, anti-inflammatory, antiseptic, antiviral, emmenagogue, expectorant, hemostatic (controls bleeding), immune tonic, nervine, stimulant and vulnerary.

Physical: Arthritis, diarrhea, liver congestion, menstrual issues, neuralgia, respiratory issues, skin sores and wounds.

Mental: Anxiety, awareness, creativity, depression, exhaustion, insomnia, motivation, nervousness, sluggish and spiritual openness.

Emotional: Bitterness, courage, emotional coldness, fear, feeling empty, frightened, intuition, passion, powerless, repressed memories and warms the heart.

Chakra: 1st (root), 3rd (solar plexus), 4th (heart), 5th (throat)

History: Some believe that Cistus is the biblical Rose of Sharon. It has been used historically in ancient perfumes and fumigation products.

Personal Experience: I use this essential oil to enhance respiration, decongest ear, nose and throat passageways, post-nasal drip and liver congestion. Emotionally it has inspired creativity, motivation, self- awareness to be in the moment as well as help with goal setting. I find it nourishes and warms the heart with a sense of courageous stamina.

Contraindications: Non-irritating.

Citronella *(Cymbopogon nardus)*

Scent: Fresh, lemony-woodsy-green scent with equal hints of sweet and earth

Note: Middle 5

Extraction Method: Steam Distillation

Parts Used: Grass and leaves

Plant Description: It is a perennial tropical grass that looks similar to lemongrass, with long leaves that grow out then flop to the side. It can grow up to 5 feet and requires hydration in moist, sandy, semi-drained soil. It thrives best in full sunlight to semi-shade (a couple hours a day). It does not like cool, damp weather. It is a member of the Gramineae family.

Chemistry: Monoterpenols (geraniol, citronellol, borneol); Phenols (methyl ether, methyl isoeugenol, isoeugenol); Monoterpenes (limonene, camphene); Aldehydes (citronellal); and Esters (geranyl acetate).

Main Body Systems: Circulatory, structural, urinary

Properties: Analgesic, antibacterial, antifungal, anti-infectious, anti-inflammatory, antiseptic, decongestant, deodorant, diaphoretic, febrifuge, insecticide, stimulant, tonic and vermifuge.

Physical: Acne, arthritis, calms rapid heartbeat, circulatory weakness, colds and flu, coughs (wet), headache, insect repellant, intestinal parasites, muscle aches and pains, neuralgia, oily skin, respiratory and breathing support, rheumatism and urinary issues.

Mental: Anxiety, communication skills, confidence, depression, fatigue, headaches, lift mood, memory, mental acuity and clarity, open-mindedness, repels "people pests" and stress.

Emotional: Anger, emotionally drained, emotional pain, feeling attacked, grief, lifts spirits, personal identity, resentment, self-doubt and strengthen personal power.

Chakra: 1ˢᵗ (root), 5ᵗʰ (throat), 6ᵗʰ (third eye)

History: Commonly used in ancient cultures for fever, intestinal parasites and digestion. In Asia, it is popular in perfumes, bug repellents, soaps and candles. Traditional Chinese Medicine uses it for rheumatic pain and in Mozambique, it is mixed in milk to strengthen blood and the nervous system. It is sometimes referred to in India as "The Oil of Tranquility," because it supports achieving wisdom and a deeper connection with the higher self.

Personal Experience: I use this essential oil as an insect repellent, for insect bites, fevers, oily skin and joint pain. Emotionally, I find it opening and freeing to let the mind wander and dream with confidence and certainty.

Contraindications: May cause irritation to those with highly-sensitive skin.

Clary Sage *(Salvia sclarea)*

Scent: Earthy, sweet, clean, airy, warming, tea-like

Note: Middle

Extraction Method: Steam Distillation

Parts Used: Flowers and/or leaves

Plant Description: It is a biennial and perennial plant that can grow up to 3 feet high. It has large, heart-shaped leaves with purple and white flowers that grow in tall clusters with pointed tips. It prefers dry, well-drained, acidic soil in the sunlight as it does not grow well in the shade. It is a member of the Labiatae family.

Chemistry: Esters (linalyl acetate, geranyl acetate, neryl acetate); Monoterpenols (linalool, geraniol); Sesquiterpenes (germacrene, caryophyllene); Diterpenols (sclareol);Monoterpenes (myrcene); Oxides (1,8 cineole, caryophyllene oxide); Ketones (thujone); Sesquiterpinols; Aldehydes; and Coumarins.

Main Body Systems: Circulatory (cephalic), glandular, nervous

Properties: Analgesic, antibacterial, antidepressant, antigalactagogue, antispasmodic, antiviral, aphrodisiac, carminative, emmenagogue, euphoric, hypotensive, nervine and sedative.

Physical: Alopecia, asthma, fibromyalgia, hemorrhoids, hormone balance, improve vision, lower blood pressure, menopause, muscle pain and spasms, neuralgia, PMS cramps, sciatica, heart tonic and urinary concerns.

Mental: Anxiety, compulsive, confidence, creativity, hysteria, indecision, jealous, mental blocks, mental clarity and vision, mood swings, obsessive, phobias, PTSD, racing thoughts and stress.

Emotional: Emotional cleansing, emotionally cold, withdrawn and confused, frustration, happiness, hysteria, irritable, joy, past emotional wounds, paranoid, pleasure, rage, sadness, trauma and unconditional love of self.

Chakra: 1ˢᵗ (root), 2ⁿᵈ (sacral), 4ᵗʰ (heart), 6ᵗʰ (third eye), 7ᵗʰ (crown)

History: Clary sage was commonly used in ancient cultures for perfumes, deodorants, soaps and skin care. Noted often for its emmenagogue properties and nervine benefits, Europe employs it for menopausal discomfort, menstrual pain and regulation. Germans use the seeds as a flavor enhancer for muscatel wine.

Personal Experience: I like to use this essential oil for nerve and muscle pain, PMS cramps, menopause discomfort, cold emotions, to lift mood and promote laughter. I add one drop to my facial sauna when clearing the pores, promoting creativity and visioning and to strengthen eye health.

Contraindications: Do not use with people with estrogen-dominant cancers. Avoid over-stimulation as it can enhance vivid dreams and possibly nightmares.

✓ Clove *(Eugenia caryophyllata)*

Scent: Spicy, heating, drying, stimulating, pungent with camphor undertones

Note: Middle 6

Extraction Method: Steam Distillation

Parts Used: Bud (unripe), leaves, stems

Plant Description: It is an evergreen tree that can grow to a height 30 feet. The entire tree is aromatic with a pyramidal shape. The glossy green leaves grow on long, slender branches with varied colored flowers buds through maturity that produce small, oblong berries. It prefers wet, semi-drained, sandy soil and in warm temperatures. It is a member of the Myrtaceae family.

Chemistry: Phenols (eugenol); Esters (eugenyl acetate); Sesquiterpenes (caryophyllene, humulene); Oxides (caryophyllene oxide); Carboxylic Acids; and Ketones.

Main Body Systems: Gastrointestinal, immune, nervous

Properties: Analgesic, antiparasitic, anti-infectious, antiviral, antibacterial, antifungal, antiseptic, antispasmodic, aphrodisiac, carminative, expectorant, stimulant and vermifuge.

Physical: Arthritis, exhaustion, immune strength, intestinal parasites, nervousness, neuralgia, pain, pulmonary concerns, ringworm, rheumatism, sciatica and toothaches.

Mental: Addictions, amnesia, anxiety, creativity, intellectual weakness, lethargy, memory, mental stimulation, mental fatigue, quiets negative thoughts, sleepiness, stress and worry.

Emotional: Cleanses the aura, connect to self-awareness, contentment, emotional sluggishness that allows for invasion of personal space, inspiration and passion, and warms cold emotions.

Chakra: 1st (root), 2nd (sacral), 5th (throat), 6th (third eye), 7th (crown)

History: Used during the war to disinfect hospitals and treat battle wounds. Considered by ancient physicians to ward off disease and plague. Romans use for headaches, hearing, chilliness and dropsy (edema). Used in numerous cultural culinary dishes, and a popular remedy to relieve toothaches and combat gum infections. Ayurveda and Chinese medicine use in muscle and nerve atrophy.

Personal Experience: I use this essential oil to disinfect the air and surfaces, combat illness, pain and neuralgia, aid in digestion and intestinal parasites, stimulate mental circulation and in a flea and ant repellent. Emotionally it warms cold emotions, opening the heart and mind.

Contraindications: Avoid during pregnancy. May inhibit blood clotting so avoid with blood thinners with slow blood clotting. May be irritating to liver if over-exposure for long periods of time. Known skin irritant, especially when undiluted.

✓ Coriander *(Coriandrum sativum)*

Scent: Fresh, green, clean with earthy, dry and semi-sweet undertones

Note: Middle 5

Extraction Method: Steam distillation

Parts used: Seeds

Plant Description: It is an annual herbal plant that can grow up to 3 feet tall. It has a tall, slender stalk with dark, rich green, feathery leaflets (cilantro). It produces tiny white to pink flowers that turn into small, ribbed, brownish-yellow seeds (coriander) that have a strong odor (becomes better when it is dried). It prefers dry, well-drained, alkaline soil in shaded to semi-shaded areas. It is a member of the Umbelliferae family. This plant also produces coriander which is distilled from the seeds.

Chemistry: Monoterpenols (linalool, coriandrol, geraniol, borneol); Mono-terpenes (pinene, terpinene, limonene, cymene); Esters (geranyl acetate, linalyl acetate); Ketones (camphor, carvone); Aldehyde (decyl aldehyde); and Ethers (anethole).

Main Body Systems: Digestive, nervous, urinary

Properties: Antibacterial, antifungal, anti-halitosis, antispasmodic, antiviral, aphrodisiac carminative, depurative, expectorant, febrifuge, narcotic, stimulant and stomachic.

Physical: Arthritis, colds, digestive aid, ease childbirth and associated pain, gastrointestinal spasms, gout, nausea, neuralgia, oily skin and blackheads, PMS, urinary support.

Mental: Depression, dizziness, fatigue, headache, insomnia, memory recall, mental clarity, motivation, nervous, post-partum depression, secretive and stress.

Emotional: Anger, bitterness, disconnectedness, fear, hopeful, insecure, joy, laughter, pessimism, refreshed, rejuvenated, self-confidence, shock, undernourished and worry.

Chakra: 1st (root), 2nd (sacral), 4th (heart), 5th (throat) and 6th (third eye)

History: The Egyptians believed it to possess the secret to happiness and were used at funerals in the Egyptian tombs. Greek and Romans used it as a medicine to preserve foods, stimulate digestion and calm nerves. Coriander is also employed extensively as a flavoring for gin, and other alcoholic liquors.

Personal Experience: I use this essential oil to balance sebum on skin, combat blackheads and oily skin. It also helps balance blood sugar and stimulate digestion. Emotionally, I find it purifying, refreshing and rejuvenating.

Contraindications: Use sparingly with chronic asthma. Can have narcotic effect in high amounts.

Cypress *(Cupressus sempervirens)*

Scent: Woodsy, earth, green scent, hints of spice, clean, refreshing

Note: Base 8

Extraction Method: Steam Distillation

Parts Used: Needles, leaf, bark

Plant Description: It is an evergreen tree that can grow up to 150 feet high. It has tiny, coarse, bristle-like leaves on strong, slender branches that contribute to its pyramidal shape. It produces small, round cones. It prefers sandy, well-drained soil in warm, sunny climates and is drought tolerant. It cannot grow in the shade. It is a member of the Cupressaceae family.

Properties: Antibacterial, antiseptic, antiviral, antispasmodic, astringent, expectorant, diuretic, hepatic, hemostatic, lymphatic drainage, styptic, sudorific and tonic.

Chemistry: Monoterpenes (pinene, 3-carene, limonene, terpinolene, cymene); Sesquiterpenols (cedrol); Monoterpenols (borneol, terpineol, sabinol); Esters (terpinyl acetate); Sesquiterpenes (cadinene, cedrene); Diterpenols; and Oxides.

Main Body Systems: Circulatory, lymphatic, urinary

Physical: Bedwetting, cellulite, enhances circulation, congested skin, incontinence, lymphatic stagnation, osteoarthritis, PMS pain and regulation, respiratory concerns, right-sided issues, rosacea, urinary issues and vein health.

Mental: Alertness, anger, anxiety, clarity, concentration, creativity, depression, forgetful, inner knowing, mental sluggishness, mood swings, nervousness, PTSD, stress and trauma.

Emotional: Emotional strength, grief (death and loss), grounding, irritability, nurturing, relationship struggles with father or father-figure, supports during times of transition (death, new location or career, puberty, menopause), sadness, self-doubt, self-worth and spiritual connection.

Chakra: 1st (root), 2nd (sacral), 4th (heart), 5th (throat), 6th (third eye)

History: A popular tree in cemeteries among the Egyptians, as they dedicated it to their Gods of the underworld. Greeks used to make statues of Gods, heroes and authorities. Phoenicians and Cretans built houses and ships, as the wood is very strong and durable. Hippocrates used it to arrest bleeding and for hemorrhoids, gum and internal bleeding. Dr. Jean Valnet used with patients for bronchitis.

Personal Experience: I use this essential oil to stimulate circulation, decongest the lymph, combat cellulite, rosacea and for vein support. Emotionally it is grounding, keeping my feet on the earth and stabilizing while being flexible.

Contraindications: Non-irritating.

Davana (*Artemisia pallens*)

Scent: Rich, sweet, woody-herbaceous scent with pungent, balsamic undertones

Note: Base 7-8

Extraction Method: Steam Distillation

Parts Used: Leaves and flowers

Plant Description: It is a perennial plant that can grow up to 2 feet high. It has snowflake-shaped, green leaves on succulent stems and produces small, sponge-like yellow flowers. It prefers dry climates in full sunlight with dry, acidic soil. It inhibits other plants grown around it, so it can control its area. It is a member of the Compositae family.

Properties: Antibacterial, antifungal, antiparasitic, antiseptic, antispasmodic, antiviral, aphrodisiac, emmenagogue, expectorant, insecticide, mucolytic, nervine, sedative and vulnerary.

Chemistry: Ketones (davanone, nordavanone); Ethers (davana ether); and Furanoids (davana furan).

Main Body Systems: Glandular, nervous, respiratory

Physical: Adrenal exhaustion, cold and flu, diabetes, dry skin, high blood pressure, muscle spasms, neuro-endocrine system support, respiratory distress, thyroid and urinary issues.

Mental: Anxiety, courage, creativity, depression, fatigue, inner strength, insomnia, mental chaos, mental clarity, nervous tension, positive thoughts, refreshes the mind, shock and stress.

Emotional: Anger, betrayal, deep-seated emotions, deter "people pests", disappointment, emotional trauma recovery, enhances intuition and inner peace, grounding, jealousy, PTSD, supports during transformations.

Chakra: 1st (root), 5th (throat), 6th (third eye)

History: In India the blossoms are used as an offering to Shiva. Ayurveda medicine uses it to reduce blood glucose in diabetics, address mental health issues, nervousness, coughs and more. It is commonly used in perfumes, past and present.

Personal Experience: I use this essential oil to promote a deeper, grounding spiritual awareness and connection with myself, encourage self-love and overcome feeling of being defeated. It helps promote clear, positive thoughts to minimize PTSD feelings. Great to enhance breathing and get a good night's rest.

Contraindications: Use caution during pregnancy due to its emmenagogue properties. Use sparingly with epilepsy, children and pets due to its high ketone content.

Dill (*Anethum graveolens*)

Scent: Green, herbaceous with sweet, camphor, earth and mint undertones

Note: Middle 5-6

Extraction Method: Steam Distillation

Parts Used: Leaves

Plant Description: It is an annual herbal plant that can grow up to 2 feet tall. Its leaves are feathery and fern-like with yellow flowers that look like a firework. It grows best in damp soil in full sunlight, as it does not thrive in the shade. It is a member of the Umbelliferae family.

Properties: Anti-anxiety, antibacterial, antidepressant, antispasmodic, antiviral, carminative, digestive, diuretic, galactagogue, stomachic and tonic.

Chemistry: Monoterpenes (limonene, pinene, phellandrene); Ketones (carvone); Ethers (dill ether); Coumarins; and Furanocoumarins.

Main Body Systems: Digestive, nervous, urinary

Physical: Bone strength, colic, digestive upset, dry conditions (skin, mouth, lungs), intestinal spasms, kidney support, pain and swelling, respiratory issues and urinary tract concerns.

Mental: Concentration, confidence, confusion, creativity, determination, enhance wit, headache, insomnia, mental chatter, mental stamina, mental suppression, moody and nervousness.

Emotional: Courage, disappointment, emotional conflict, emotional dryness and dehydration, hypersensitive to criticism, irritable, not speaking up for self, overwhelmed, sadness and worry.

Chakra: 1st (root), 2nd (sacral), 7th (crown)

History: Used often in Europe, Mediterranean and West African regions in culinary dishes for its medicinal properties. It is referenced in the Bible and in ancient Egyptian writings. Hippocrates used it for cleaning the mouth. Ancient soldiers would apply dill seeds to their wounds to promote healing. Greek and Roman warriors would spread it all over their body for a muscle toner.

Personal Experience: I use this essential oil for digestive upset, muscle pain relief and to inspire mood. Emotionally it has infused positivity when I am feeling down and disappointed.

Contraindications: Use caution during pregnancy.

Elemi *(Canarium luzonicum)*

Scent: Herbaceous, green scent with peppery, balsamic and bitter undertones

Note: Middle to Top Base 7-8

Extraction Method: Steam Distillation

Parts Used: Resin

Plant Description: It is a large, deciduous tree that can grow as tall as 90 feet high. Many leaflets cover the branches that spread out to the sides, and produce green-yellow clusters of flowers and a hard nut or fruit that turns from green to deep blue-purple when ripe. The thick resin that exudes from the tree bark, is used for distillation. It requires lots of rainfall and moisture, and can grow best in deep, fertile, well-drained soil. It does not like cool temperatures or frost but can survive hurricanes and typhoons. It is a member of the Burseraceae family.

Chemistry: Monoterpenes (limonene, phellandrene, sabinene); Sesquiterpenols (elemol); Ethers (elemicin); Sesquiterpenes (elemene); Monoterpinols; and Ketones.

Main Body Systems: Immune, respiratory, structural

Properties: Anti-allergenic, antibacterial, antifungal, anti-inflammatory, antiseptic, cicatrisant, expectorant, febrifuge, stomachic, stimulant, tonic and vulnerary.

Physical: Asthma, bone repair and strength, bronchitis, colds and flu, combats airborne pathogens, dry cough, immunity, muscle tension and spasms, pneumonia and skin support (mature, wrinkles, irritations, rashes, scars).

Mental: Adjust to changes (wrap your head around it), anxiety, conquer new visions and tasks with spunk, creative zest, depression, determination, grounding, mediation, mental fatigue, nervousness, positive thinking and stress.

Emotional: Compassion, contentment, deep emotional wounds, encourage calmness, feels like you are being punished or want to punish others, grief, helps one weather the storm, promotes peace and a tranquil heart, restoration during chaos, revitalizing and trauma warrior.

Chakra: It balances the upper and lower chakras.

History: It was first cultivated in the ancient Philippines as an edible fruit. Egyptians used it for embalming and preservative properties. Being a strong base not and fixative, it was used often in perfumes. In 16th century Europe the resin was used for ulcers, skin irritations, broken bones, battle wounds and head traumas of soldiers, as it accelerated healing. It has a reputation of being a "poor man's frankincense".

Personal Experience: I use this essential oil to boost immunity and ward off germs, especially when I travel, and to strengthen breathing and respiratory functions. I've also used it in bone and wound salves, acne toners and skin irritation creams.

Contraindications: Non-irritating.

Eucalyptus *(Eucalyptus globulus)*

Scent: Camphoraceous, pungent, penetrating, fresh, slightly sweet scent

Note: Middle 6-7

Extraction Method: Steam Distillation

Parts Used: Leaves and twigs

Plant Description: There are many varieties of eucalyptus. They are the tallest evergreen trees and have been noted to reach heights of 480 feet. It has with glossy green or waxy silver-green leaves (covered in tiny oil glands) that produces varied colored flowers with hair-like petals and nuts. The branches and trunks are flexible but durable and rot-resistant. It prefers warm weather with moist but well-drained soil and sunlight. All eucalyptus is in the Myrtaceae family.

Properties: Analgesic, antibacterial, antifungal, antiseptic, antispasmodic, antiviral, decongestant, expectorant, febrifuge, insecticide, stimulant, sudorific and tonic.

Chemistry: Oxides (1,8 cineole): Monoterpenes (pinene, limonene, cymene); Sesquiterpenols (globulol, pinocarveol); Sesquiterpenes (aromadendrene); Ketones (pinocarvone); Aldehydes; Phenols (myrtenol); Monoterpenols (fenchol, terpin-4-ol); and Esters.

Main Body Systems: Immune, respiratory, structural

Physical: Air purifier, cold and flu, cold sores, coughs, decongestant, deodorant, diabetes, fevers, gingivitis, insect repellant, open nasal passageways to relieve congestion, respiratory issues (bronchitis, pneumonia), sinus infections, sore muscles and urinary issues.

Mental: Addictions, calm nit-picking, clears and opens the mind, concentration, creativity, focus, headaches, memory recall, mental chatter, mentally suffocated and constrictions, obsessions, refreshes thoughts and self-confidence.

Emotional: Balances the head and heart, bitterness, blame, desire to run, emotionally stagnant, overwhelmed, guilt, hostility, move forward, need room to breathe, protects from pestering people, resentment, self-esteem and smothered.

Chakra: 4th (heart), 5th (throat), 6th (third eye), 7th (crown)

History: Known to be the main food for koalas in Australia. It was noted as early as the 1880s, that surgeons used it as an antiseptic during operations. In ancient times, it was used as a tea for fevers, colds, coughs and immune distress. In 19th century England, it was used in hospitals to clean urinary catheters. Sicilians planted to combat malaria. The wood burns fast in a fire, thus "eucalyptus type" people do not do well if they have been "burned". Eucalyptus globulus is one of the most studied of this species and most medicinal.

Personal Experience: I use this essential oil for a variety of reasons from respiratory expectorant and decongestant, coughs, colds, muscle aches and pains to opening my mind when I am brainstorming, or too focused on a situation. It gives me room to breathe with a fresh, positive outlook.

Contraindications: Use caution with epilepsy and asthma. May cause skin irritations. Check with pharmacists for possible prescription interactions.

Other species: *Eucalyptus radiata; smithii; citriodora*

> **Eucalyptus citriodora**: Does not grow as tall as *Eucalyptus globulus*. It more lemony, peppery floral scent thus it is more preferred in the perfume industry. Its nickname is "lemon-scented eucalyptus". This is the one I prefer in my flea, tick and bug repellent.

> **Eucalyptus radiata**: Does not grow as tall as *Eucalyptus globulus*. This has a more pepperminty scent, hence its nickname, "peppermint eucalyptus". Used more interchangeably with globulus for expectorant and decongestant properties.

> **Eucalyptus smithii**: Does not grow as tall as *Eucalyptus globulus* and has a milder, earthier scent.

Fennel *(foeniculum vulgare; var. dulse, amara)*

Scent: Rich, licorice scent with spicy, sweet camphor undertones

Note: Middle 7

Extraction Method: Steam Distillation

Parts Used: Seeds

Plant Description: It is a perennial plant that can grow up to 5 feet tall. It has a strong root bulb, dark green, feathery leaves and yellow flowers that look like mini fireworks. The flowers produce brown, silvery-green seeds. It prefers dry, acid soil in direct sunlight. It does not like the shade and is drought tolerant. It is a member of the Umbelliferae family.

Properties: Antibacterial, antispasmodic, antiseptic, antiviral, carminative, diaphoretic, digestive, diuretic, emmenagogue, expectorant, galactagogue, hepatic, stimulant, stomachic and vermifuge.

Chemistry: Ethers (anethole, estragole); Monoterpenes (ocimene, limonene, terpinene, pinene, phellandrene); Monoterpenols (linalool, fenchol); Ketones (fenchone); Oxides (1,8 cineole); Phenols; Furanocoumarins; and Coumarins.

Main Body Systems: Digestion, intestinal, urinary

Physical: Colic, coughs, cramps and spasms, edema, enhance detoxification and elimination, eyesight strength, gum support, indigestion, kidney and bladder concerns, liver and lymphatic congestion, nausea and respiratory and breathing concerns.

Mental: Anxiety, clear thinking, insomnia, mental endurance, over think and analysis, releasing creative blocks, renewing interest in life and sluggish cognitive functions.

Emotional: Connect to inner wisdom, courage, emotional resilience and strength, emotional repression, helps digest a situation and adapt to the changes, nervous tension, recover from "snake-like people" attacks, self-esteem and shed the past to open yourself up to the new.

Chakra: 1st (root), 3rd (solar plexus), 4th (heart), 5th (throat), 7th (crown)

History: Egyptians and Hippocrates used medicinally for several purposes. Romans used it often in culinary dishes as it helped with digestion and other functions. Greeks knew it by the name "marathon", as it grew in the field in which one of the great ancient battles was fought and named the Battle of Marathon after this revered plant. Historically, ancient physicians and herbalist have associated it with eye health such as cataracts and blindness, as well as to neutralize the poison of snake bites.

Personal Experience: I use this essential oil to help with digestive issues such as gas, bloating and indigestion. It also helps bring clarity to the "gut brain" and helps it communicate better with the "head brain", hence mental clarity and focus. I also like it to support kidney, lymphatic and liver elimination. Emotionally I find it gives me a resilience to endure tough situations.

Contraindications: Avoid with epilepsy, liver disease and certain pulmonary concerns. It can be irritating to the skin and membranes. Not for ingestion.

Firs

There are many fir species, and several that are essential oils. Firs are hearty, woody, opening, simultaneously refreshing and grounding, durable and help one connect to themselves on a deeper level with clarity and acceptance. They are the most popular choice for a Christmas tree and timber in the USA.

Balsam Fir (*Abies balsamea*)

Scent: Woody, green, rich earth scent with hearty balsamic and sweet undertones

Note: Middle to base 7-8

Extraction Method: Steam Distillation

Parts Used: Needles, leaves, branches

Plant Description: It is a pyramidal shaped evergreen tree that can reach heights of 65-90 feet. It has soft, thin resinous but durable branches, green, bristle-like needle leaves and dark brown-purple cones that stay closed up until time to release the seeds. It prefers moist, acid soil in shaded to semi-shaded areas, but can tolerate sunlight but not wind, due to its shallow roots. It is a member of the Pinaceae family.

Properties: Analgesic, antibacterial, antifungal, anti-inflammatory, antiseptic, antispasmodic, diuretic, febrifuge, insecticide, mucolytic, stimulant and vulnerary.

Chemistry: Monoterpenes (pinene, phellandrene, limonene, 3-carene, myrcene, camphene); Esters (bornyl acetate); Monoterpenols (linalool, terpineol); and Sesquiterpenes (bisabolene, longifolene, caryophyllene, humulene) *(http://www.sciencedirect.com/science/article/pii/S0031942200912901)*.

Main Body Systems: Nervous, respiratory, urinary

Physical: Arthritis, burns, coughs, fever, increases metabolism, joint pain, nerve pain, reduces body odor, respiratory congestion, sore muscles, sore throats and wounds.

Mental: Anxiety, calming, clear thoughts, concentration, fatigue, grounding, insomnia, mental exhaustion, headache, relaxation and visioning clarity.

Emotional: Anger, dominance, feel you easily get burned, fear, grief, guilt, inner peace, irritation, self-acceptance, stability, thriving under someone's shadow and weeping.

Chakra: 1st (root), 3rd (solar plexus), 5th (throat), 6th (third eye)

History: Native Americans used it for various medicinal uses. Tribes made a tea from the sap or bark, and smelled the burning wood for respiratory concerns. A balm of balsam fir resin was used during Civil War as an external application to the injuries of combat. It serves as a source of food for various animals. Its oleoresin is often used to help mount microscopic specimens and serves as a cement for various parts of optical systems.

Personal Experience: I use this essential oil to promote a sense of grounding, keeping me connected to the earth and my instincts. It helps during times of being dominated or domineering, feeling uneasy with thoughts and gut, emotional stability and skin traumas such as cuts, burns and rashes.

Contraindications: Non-irritating.

Douglas-Fir (*Pseudotsuga menziesii*)

Scent: Rich, green, woody, balsamic-earth scent with slight camphoraceous, dry undertones

Note: Middle to base 7-8

Extraction Method: Steam Distillation

Parts Used: Needles, leaves, branches

Plant Description: It is a pyramidal shaped evergreen conifer tree that can reach heights of 300 feet. The bark on the trunk gets thicker with age and has strong, wind-resistant branches. It has dark, silvery-green needles that are bristle-like, and the cones scales fold up in layers similar to a rose. It prefers deep, wet but well-drained loamy soil, with lots of moisture and sunlight. It cannot grow in the shade and is not frost sensitive. It is a member of the Pinaceae family.

Properties: Antibacterial, antifungal, anti-rheumatic, antiseptic, digestive, emmenagogue, expectorant, sedative, tonic and vulnerary.

Chemistry: Monoterpenes (pinene, limonene, 3-carene); Esters (bornyl acetate, geranyl acetate); Monoterpenols (borneol, geraniol, linalool); Sesquiterpenes (longifolene); and Aldehydes.

Main Body Systems: Digestion, respiratory, structural

Physical: Adrenal support, athlete's foot, bone health (broken or dislocated), colds and flu, coughs, digestive upset, joint pain, kidney and bladder concerns, nausea, PMS, rosacea, respiratory concerns, skin issues, sore throat and wounds.

Mental: Alert, anxiety, creative dreams and goal-setting, dizzy, grounding, mental chatter, mental congestion, nervousness, opens and refreshes the mind, perfectionist, relaxation and sleepiness.

Emotional: Anger, contentment, fear of failure, frustration with being so dutiful, guilt, peaceful, self-awareness and acceptance, sensitive to criticism, stable in times of chaos and confusion, suppressed and vivacious.

Chakra: 1st (root), 4th (heart)

History: Douglas-fir has had a tough time being classified. Although it has some similar characteristics and genetic material, it is not actually a pine, spruce or true fir, hence the hyphen. It is the state tree of Oregon, USA and it often referred to as "Oregon pine" or Douglas spruce. It got its common name, *Douglas-fir*, from the Scottish botanist David Douglas who introduced many native North American conifers to Europe, and in 1826 introduced *Pseudotsuga menziesii* into cultivation. Native Americans burned it as fuel and to make fishing hooks, harpoon shafts and handles for fishing nets. It is the second largest conifer (after redwoods) in the world. It is one of the most popular choices in the USA for a Christmas tree.

Personal Experience: I use this essential oil to ground my mind, helping me get centered and to accept and love myself. It brings me deep contentment within. Physically I like it to support my adrenals, nerves and urinary system.

Contraindications: Non-irritating.

Himalayan Fir (*Abies spectabilis*)

Scent: Woody, green scent with slight camphoraceous, wet, earthy undertones

Note: Middle to base 7-8

Extraction Method: Steam Distillation

Parts Used: Needles, leaves, branches

Plant Description: It is a pyramidal shaped evergreen coniferous tree that can reach heights of 180 feet. Its reddish-brown branches grow out horizontally, has dark, silvery-green, glossy needles that are bristle like with cones that turn from purple to dark brown as they mature. It prefers heavy clay, moist, acid soil grown in full shade or no shade. It is frost sensitive. It is a member of the Pinaceae family.

Properties: Analgesic, anti-inflammatory, antiseptic, carminative, disinfectant, expectorant, sedative, stomachic, tonic and vulnerary.

Chemistry: Monoterpenes (pinene, santene, limonene, camphene); Esters (bornyl acetate); Diterpenes; Triterpenes; and Phenols.

Main Body Systems: Nervous, respiratory, urinary

Physical: Adrenal support, arthritis, deodorant, immune support, kidney and urinary support, muscle pain and soreness, respiratory concerns, sinus issues, skin irritations and thyroid support.

Mental: Anxiety, concentration, exhaustion, focus, headache, high blood pressure, insomnia, mental stillness, migraines, nervousness, repetitive thoughts, speaking up for self and vitality.

Emotional: Anger, courage, cools a heated heart, emotional cleansing of negativity and chaos, emotionally cold, feel like you are missing something, let go of grudges and past trauma, oppressed and yearning to travel.

Chakra: 1st (root, 2nd (sacral), 4th (heart), 5th (throat), 7th (crown)

History: It has been used to make incense sticks, furniture and firewood. The leaf juice has been used for asthma and bronchitis. Used often to strengthen lung function.

Personal Experience: I use this essential oil for respiratory and urinary concerns. Emotionally, it gives me room to breathe without feeling constrained or closed in. It helps me feel a deeper connection to self and the earth, grounded and relaxed.

Contraindications: Non-irritating.

Siberian Fir *(Abies siberica)*

Scent: Woody, green scent with slight camphor, earthy undertones

Note: Middle to base 7-8

Extraction Method: Steam Distillation

Parts Used: Needles, leaves, branches

Plant Description: It is a pyramidal shaped evergreen conifer tree that can reach heights of 100 feet. It has strong branches that grows out and slightly upward, green-grey needle leaves and purple to dark brown cones. It prefers heavy clay, moist, acid soil grown in full shade or no shade. It is frost resistant, and rarely lives over 200 years old if exposed to fungus. It is a member of the Pinaceae family.

Chemistry: Monoterpenes (camphene, pinene, terpinene, limonene); Esters (bornyl acetate, terpinyl acetate); Monoterpenols (borneol, terpineol); and Sesquiterpenes (bisabolene, caryophyllene) *(http://link.springer.com/article/10.1007%2Fs11094-014-1131-6#/page-1)*.

Main Body Systems: Immune, respiratory, urinary

Properties: Analgesic, antibacterial, anti-inflammatory, antifungal, anti-rheumatic, antiseptic, antispasmodic, decongestant, expectorant and stimulant.

Physical: Arthritis, circulation, colds and flu, digestive aid, immune support, muscle recovery, pain, respiratory concerns, swelling, thrush and ulcers.

Mental: Anxiety, clear intentions, confidence, inspires motivation, lifts mood and spirit, move forward without fear, positive thoughts, restores vital energy and self-doubt.

Emotional: Anger, acceptance and understanding, contentment, feel connected to self, feel defeated, frustration, intolerance of toxic relationships, joy, love of self, overwhelmed, sadness, smothered and supports during times of transition.

Chakra: 3rd (solar plexus) 4th (heart), 5th (throat), 6th (third eye)

History: Firs are known for their strength. The wood is soft, lightweight and weak making it good to build furniture. They built ships with it in 17th century Europe. Commonly used in muscle rubs, respiratory decongestants and perfumes.

Personal Experience: I use this essential oil for grounding, relaxation, quiet mental chatter, self-love and joy, immune support and in a bath salt for muscle pain. It gives a sense of deeper connection and stillness.

Contraindications: Use caution with severe pulmonary issues and asthma.

Silver Fir (*Abies alba*)

Scent: Green, woody scent with slight camphoraceous, airy but earthy undertones

Note: Middle to base 7-8

Extraction Method: Steam Distillation

Parts Used: Needles, leaves, branches

Plant Description: It is a pyramidal shaped evergreen conifer tree that can reach heights of 160-200 feet. The trunk is very thick with scaly bark and strong branches. It has dark green, glossy needle leaves that form a tight-nit bristle and the cones have scales that flare out to the side. It prefers heavy clay, moist, acid soil grown in full shade or no shade. It is frost resistant but cannot tolerate atmospheric pollution. It is a member of the Pinaceae family.

Properties: Analgesic, antibacterial, anti-rheumatic, antiseptic, astringent, diuretic, expectorant, febrifuge, immuno-stimulant, vasoconstrictor and vulnerary.

Chemistry: Monoterpenes (limonene, pinene, camphene); Esters (bornyl acetate); Monoterpinols; Diterpenols; Triterpenols; and Sesquiterpenes.

Main Body Systems: Circulatory, respiratory, urinary

Physical: Adrenal support, arthritis, bronchitis, coughs, circulator tonic, cystitis, fever, hormone balance, immune support, joint issues, nervous tension, neuropathy, respiratory distress, sinus, skin irritations and urinary concerns.

Mental: Anxiety, concentration, indecisive, grounding, impatience, insomnia, lifts mood, mental fatigue, nervousness, organize ideas and relaxing yet uplifting.

Emotional: Adapt to and balance light and dark emotions, emotional coldness, emotional freedom, fear, grief, helplessness, inner strength, inner struggle, overwhelmed, room to breathe, sadness, shyness, shock and trauma.

Chakra: 5th (throat), 6th (third eye)

History: It has been used historically for its edible inner bark in culinary dishes and soups. Commonly used for coughs, colds and rheumatism medicines, deodorants, perfumes and soaps.

Personal Experience: I use this essential oil to open my sinuses, help deepen my breathing and refresh my mind. I feel grounded and "free" to just be me. Physically, I like it for respiratory, urinary and adrenal support.

Contraindications: Non-irritating.

Frankincense *(Boswellia carteri)*

Scent: Balsamic, woody, dry, rich, intense scent

Note: Base 9-10

Extraction Method: Steam Distillation

Parts Used: Resin

Plant Description: There are four main species that produce true frankincense. It is a tree that grows up and spreads outward to about 12 feet in height with a 3-4 foot diameter trunk. It has gnarled branches with narrow, curvy-edged leaves and small clusters of white-yellow, seed-containing flowers. To obtain the essential oil from the resin, incisions are made into the trunk, the bark peeled away allowing the milky-white gum-resin tears to exude. It prefers limestone, alkaline soil in warmer climates. It is not frost tolerant. It is a member of the Burseraceae family.

Properties: Analgesic, anti-allergenic, anti-arthritic, antibacterial, anti-inflammatory, antifungal, antiseptic, antiviral, cicatrisant, diuretic, emmenagogue, expectorant, immune-stimulant, relaxant, sedative, tonic and vulnerary.

Chemistry: Monoterpenes (pinene, thujene, limonene, myrcene, sabinene); Sesquiterpenes (caryophyllene); Monoterpenols (incensol, borneol); Sesquiterpenols (farnesol, cadinene); and Diterpenes.

Main Body Systems: Immune, respiratory, structural

Physical: Acne, allergies (pet and environmental), asthma, bronchitis, dry coughs, emphysema, enhances breathing, fatigue, intestinal issues (IBS), lymph congestion (especially in breast area), nervous system relaxant and tonic, relieves heavy periods and cramping, rheumatoid arthritis, skin concerns (mature, wrinkles, scars, dryness, burns) and urinary concerns.

Mental: Anxiety, creativity, concentration, confusion, depression, indecision, insomnia, inspiration, meditation, mental chatter, mental clarity, nervous tension, nightmares, over-thinking, purify the aura, restless, self-awareness and discipline, spiritual aid, strengthens faith and stress.

Emotional: Acceptance, anger, contentment, courage, disconnected to inner soul, feel defeated, grief, guilt, grounding, hopeful, irritability, jealousy, panic and out of control, promotes understanding, quarrelsome, relieves fear and fright, self-worth, sorrow, withstand violent situations and worry.

Chakra: 1st (root), 4th (heart), 5th (throat), 6th (third eye), 7th (crown)

History: Most noted as a gift to the Magi, and more prized than gold. Kohl, the black powder used as eyeliner by Egyptians, was made from charred frankincense. It was used in the embalming process. Actually, scents of frankincense were still lingering when King Tut's tomb was opened in 1922. The Greeks and Romans used it often as incense offered to their gods, in religious ceremonies and hemorrhoids. Chinese Traditional Medicine used to promote the movement of blood and chi.

Personal Experience: I use this essential oil for many things. I like to add 1 drop to my facial steamer to nourish my skin but also my sinuses. It works great to calm most allergies, fear, nightmares, snoring and urinary concerns. It makes me feel grounded, supported, strong, inspired, connected and content. It also serves as a great base note in perfumes.

Contraindications: Non-irritating.

Galbanum *(Ferula galbaniflua, gummosa)*

Scent: Rich, earth, green, dirt-like with dry, slight-bitter and balsamic undertones

Note: Base 10

Extraction Method: Steam Distillation

Parts Used: Resin

Plant Description: Galbanum is a small plant that can grow up to five feet. It has glossy, serrated leaves with small clusters of yellowish flowers that look like mini fireworks, to form a big firework. The essential oil comes from resin ducts in the stems and roots. It prefers well-drained, acidic soil in the sun, as it does not grow in the shade. It is a member of the Umbelliferae family.

Properties: Antibacterial, anti-inflammatory, antispasmodic, carminative, edema, expectorant, insecticide, mucolytic, sedative, stimulant, tonic and vulnerary.

Chemistry: Monoterpenes (pinene, 3-carene, myrcene, sabinene); Sesquiterpenols (galbanol, bulnesol); Esters (fenchyl acetate, linalyl acetate); Coumarins; Furanoids; and Carboxylic Acids.

Main Body Systems: Digestion, nervous, respiratory

Physical: Arthritis, boils, circulation, digestive upset, epilepsy, hemorrhoids, hot flashes, libido support, lymphatic congestions, muscle soreness, PMS issues, respiratory issues and skin issues (acne, mature, wrinkles, scars).

Mental: Agoraphobia, anxiety, calming, claustrophobia, concentration, confidence, depression, enhances communication, grounding, hysteria, inflexible thinking, intuition booster, nervous tension, panic, season affective disorder, stress relief and unblock buried memories.

Emotional: Acceptance and understanding of life's challenges, brings joy to the heart, eliminates emotional debris, feel confined, feel like you are kept in the dark, stabilizes emotions, struggle with emotional conflicts and traumatic wounds.

Chakra: 1st (root), 3rd (solar plexus), 5th (throat)

History: Galbanum was used as an incense in ancient civilizations. In Egypt, it was used along with Frankincense and Myrrh in baths, and in making perfume oils and cosmetics. It was used for medicinal purposes in the Middle East. Today it is more widely used in perfumes, jewelry making and as flavoring in alcoholic beverages and soft drinks.

Personal Experience: I use this essential oil as a base note in perfumes, for dry coughs, to feel grounded, connected with the earth and to help work through emotional conflicts. It helps me feel strong, confident and capable.

Contraindications: Avoid during pregnancy do to its emmenagogue properties.

Geranium *(Pelargonium graveolens)*

Scent: Floral, rose-like, sweet and earthy with slight green undertones

Note: Middle 5

Extraction Method: Steam Distillation

Parts Used: Flowers, leaf

Plant Description: It is a perennial evergreen plant that can grow almost five feet tall. It has strongly aromatic, soft, hairy, semi-serrate leaves with white, purplish pink flowers. It prefers lots of moisture and rain in well-drained, fertile soil with full sunlight, as it is cold and shade sensitive, and drought tolerant. It is a member of the Geraniaceae family.

Properties: Antibacterial, antifungal, anti-inflammatory, antispasmodic, antiviral, astringent, aphrodisiac, cytophylactic, deodorant, diuretic, emmenagogue, hepatic, immune tonic, insecticide, tonic, vermifuge and vulnerary.

Chemistry: Monoterpenols (citronellol, geraniol, linalool, nerol); Esters (citronellyl formate, geranyl formate, geranyl acetate); Ketones (isomenthone);

Sesquiterpenes (guaiadene); Aldehydes (geranial); Monoterpenes (pinene, limonene, myrcene); Sesquiterpinols; and Furanoids.

Main Body Systems: Glandular, lymphatic, urinary

Physical: Acne, breast swelling and tenderness, bruising, cellulite, circulation, edema, hormone balancing, hot flashes, insect repellent, intestinal upset, jaundice, lymphatic stimulant, menopause, night sweats, PMS and heavy periods, poor elimination and skin concerns (combination skin, stretchmarks).

Mental: Anxiety, bitterness, depression, dispels negativity, fatigue, fear, insomnia, mental clutter and stagnation, resentment, sluggish, stress, visualization, willpower and worry.

Emotional: Anger, calms and balances emotions, discouraged, frustration, grief, harmonizes head, heart and gut, lifts mood and spirit, protect against negativity, sadness, self-esteem, trouble letting go of past hurts and weeping.

Chakra: 3rd (solar plexus), 4th (heart), 6th (third eye)

History: It is commonly used to adulterate or dilute pure rose essential oil. Egyptians and Romans used as an anti-infectious and vulnerary. In Africa it was used for intestinal issues. England used it to relieve the pain from broken bones.

Personal Experience: I use this essential oil for many reasons such as hormone balance, stress relief, PMS cramps, mood swings, lymphatic decongestant and insect repellent. Emotionally it calms heated hormone emotions such as irritability and weepiness, brings balance and stability as well as overall harmony to the mind and body.

Contraindications: Use caution with estrogen-dependent cancers.

Ginger *(Zingiber officianale)*

Scent: Spicy, warm, sweet and peppery scent with pungent undertones

Note: Middle 6-7

Extraction Method: Steam Distillation

Parts Used: Root

Plant Description: It is an underground rhizome of the herbaceous perennial plant, which can grow up to four feet tall. The ginger root has a firm, striated exterior and interior. The blade-like, glossy leaves of the plant are long and slender with white-pink and yellow flowers that grow in a stalk-like arrangement. It prefers full or partial sun, with regular moisture and a well-drained, sandy soil. It is a member of the Zingiberaceae family.

Properties: Analgesic, antibacterial, antifungal, anti-inflammatory, antiparasitic, antiseptic, antispasmodic, antiviral, aphrodisiac, carminative, diaphoretic, expectorant, febrifuge, purgative, stimulant, stomachic, and tonic.

Chemistry: Sesquiterpenes (zingiberene, curcumene, sesquiphellandrene, farnesene, bisabolene); Monoterpenes (camphene, phellandrene, limonene, cymene); Monoterpenols (nonanol, citronellol, linalool, borneol); Sesquiterpenols (nerolidol, zingeberol, elemol); Ketones (heptanone); and Aldehydes.

Main Body Systems: Digestion, nervous, structural

Physical: Arthritis, bruises, cold and flu, cold extremities, digestion and nutrient assimilation, dry coughs, flexibility and mobility, fluid retention, hormone headaches, indigestion, nausea, neuropathy, pain relief, PMS cramping, sciatica and silent reflux.

Mental: Adapt to change, anxiety, creativity, debility, depression, dizzy, fainting, fatigue, grounding, memory recall, mental stimulation, nervous and physical exhaustion, restlessness, sharpens senses and willpower.

Emotional: Broken-heartedness, courage, despair, emotionally cold, feel like you've lost yourself, grief, guilt, lonely, loss of control, sadness, self-sacrifice, sorrow, speaking up for self, strength to set boundaries and stuckness.

Chakra: 1st (root), 2nd (sacral), 3rd (solar plexus), 5th (throat)

History: It has been a very popular culinary spice in most cultures for its digestive aid, antiparasitic, antispasmodic, carminative and anti-arthritic benefits, since ancient time. Marco Polo was noted for finding ginger in China. In the Middle Ages, ginger was so expensive that one pound could be used to purchase a sheep. It is often used to flavor beer and serve as a food preservative. It is used often today for its powerful anti-inflammatory properties.

Personal Experience: I use this essential oil to facilitate better digestion, alleviate intestinal upset, antiparasitic, muscle and joint pain, swelling and mix in oil that I apply to my feet to combat cold extremists. Emotionally it warms the heart to stimulate movement of stuck emotions and past hurts.

Contraindications: May cause skin irritation without a carrier. Avoid with blood-thinner medications and limit use during pregnancy.

Goldenrod *(Solidago canadensis)*

Scent: Green, herbaceous with sweet, pungent, floral undertones

Note: Middle 6-7

Extraction Method: Steam Distillation

Parts Used: Flowers

Plant Description: It is a woody perennial plant that can grow up to 7 feet tall. It has long, narrow blade-like leaves that grow upward, with rich, small, gold-yellow flowers that grow in stalk-like clusters. It has an underground rhizome root system. It prefers full sun, but can tolerate shade. It likes to be watered regularly, but in dry, well-drained, sandy soil. It is a member of the Compositae family.

Properties: Analgesic, antibacterial, antifungal, anti-infectious, anti-inflammatory, antispasmodic, antiviral, antiseptic, carminative, diaphoretic, diuretic, febrifuge, stimulant (gentle), styptic and vulnerary.

Chemistry: Monoterpenes (pinene, myrcene, limonene, sabinene); Sesquiterpenes (germacrene, longifolene, elemene); Monoterpenols (borneol); and Esters (bornyl acetate).

Main Body Systems: Hepatic, immune, urinary

Physical: Backaches (kidney region), candida, cystitis, diarrhea, digestive aid (gas, spasms), edema, fatigue, kidney cleanser and tonic, liver strengthener, nausea, periodontal issues, PMS, respiratory spasms, rheumatic pain, spleen tonic, skin trauma (burns, weepy rashes), sore throats, thrush and urinary issues.

Mental: Ambitious, concentration, confusion, depression, determined and driven, exhaustion and fatigue, fastidious, headache, insomnia, lethargy, mental sluggishness, motivated, passionate, positive thinking, objective, oversensitive and sleepiness.

Emotional: Apathy, buried anger, durability emotional attachments, fear, fright, feel the need to hide true self, freedom from ideal self-pressures, hard on self, joy, overwhelmed by duty/responsibility, quarrelsome, resilience and sadness.

Chakra: 2nd (sacral), 3rd (solar plexus), 4th (heart), 5th (throat)

History: It has been used in ancient times for many medicinal purposes. It is often referred to as *woundwort*. It was first used in the Middle East. Native Americans used the seeds in food for kidney nourishment and to relieve sore throats and toothaches. Thomas Edison was noted to use goldenrod to produce rubber, as it naturally contains a small percent in its leaves. The tires on the Model T given to him by his friend, Henry Ford, were made from goldenrod. Herbalist have used for centuries as a kidney and bladder tonic and cleanser.

Personal Experience: I use this essential oil for urinary issues, backaches (especially during PMS) and swelling and edema. Emotionally, it gives me an inner strength for determination, motivation and mental sluggishness.

Contraindications: Use caution with extreme kidney disorders.

✓Grapefruit, Pink *(Citrus paradisi)*

Scent: Sweet, citrus scent with floral and bitter undertones

Note: Top 2

Extraction Method: Cold Expression

Parts Used: Fruit rind

Plant Description: It is an evergreen tree that can grow up to 20-45 feet tall. It has dark green, glossy leaves and produces small white flowers and round, juicy fruits with strong, spongy rinds. It prefers warm climates, with sunlight and watered regularly, in well-drained, sandy soil. It is not frost tolerant. It is a member of the Rutaceae family.

Properties: Antibacterial, antidepressant, antifungal, antiparasitic, antiseptic, antiviral, cardiotonic, diuretic, immune-stimulant, sedative (mild), and stomachic.

Chemistry: Monoterpenes (limonene, pinene, sabinene, myrcene); Tetraterpenes (carotene, lycopene); Aldehydes (citral, citronellal); Furanocoumarins; Monoterpenols (linalool, terpin-4-ol, geraniol); and Esters (decyl acetate, neryl acetate).

Main Body Systems: Hepatic, lymphatic, urinary

Physical: Acne, anorexia, arteriosclerosis, bruising, cellulite, cholesterol, colds and flu, diabetes, earaches, edema, jet lag, liver and gall bladder cleanser, lymphatic drainage, metabolism, pore cleanser, skin issues, stagnation (physically and emotionally) and vein support.

Mental: Anxiety, fatigue, headache, improves mood, insomnia, inspiration, invigorating, irritability, moody, nervousness, self-doubt, sluggish cognitive function, stress, uplifting, visualization and vital energy.

Emotional: Bitterness, disappointment, emotional eating, encourages emotional movement, envious, fear, frustration, helps let go of past burdens, irritable, jealousy, resentment, self-satisfaction, stuckness and desire to be left alone (to avoid invasion).

Chakra: 2nd (sacral), 4th (heart), 6th (third eye)

History: It is a hybrid of sweet orange and pomelo, dating back to 1750 and nicknamed "the forbidden fruit", and given its botanical name in the 1830's. Often used in culinary dishes, as a flavor enhancer and weight loss aid as it boost metabolism and combats insulin resistance.

Personal Experience: I use this essential oil in lotions, bath salts and massage oils to stimulate lymphatic movement, cellulite and liver and gall bladder support. Emotionally it makes me feel rejuvenated, invigorating, uplifted, creative and free from bitterness.

Contraindications: Phototoxic. Avoid direct sunlight 9-12 hours after topical use.

√Helichrysum *(Helichrysum italicum, angustifolium)*

Scent: Earthy, warm but semi-dry, hay-like with floral, green and heady undertones

Note: Middle 6-7

Extraction Method: Steam Distillation

Parts Used: Flowers and flowering tops

Plant Description: It is an evergreen shrub that grows a little more than three feet in height. It has slender, tall leaf-like stems that emit the scent of curry, with clusters of small golden-yellow flowers that look spongy. It prefers acid, well-drained, sandy soil in the sunlight, as it cannot grow in the shade, and is drought and mild wind tolerant. It is a member of the Compositae family.

Properties: Analgesic, antibacterial, anti-inflammatory, antiseptic, antispasmodic, antiviral, choleretic, cytophylactic, expectorant, hepatic, nervine, sedative and vulnerary.

112

Chemistry: Esters (neryl acetate, neryl propionate, neryl butyrate); Ketones (italidione); Sesquiterpenes (curcumene, caryophyllene); Monoterpenes (pinene, limonene, camphene); Monoterpenols (linalool, geraniol, nerol); Oxides (1,8 cineole); and Phenols (eugenol).

Main Body Systems: Hepatic, nervous, structural

Physical: Allergies, bruising, chronic cough, circulation, hearing loss and tinnitus, liver and gallbladder congestion, nerve pain and repair, neuropathy, PMS, skin issues (burns, eczema, psoriasis, scars, rashes, wounds) and vein support.

Mental: Addictions, anxiety, confusion, headache, hopeful, indecisive, lethargy, mental chatter, mental sluggishness, negativity, nervousness, relaxing, self-doubt, self-esteem and willpower.

Emotional: Anger (repressed), bitterness, deep emotional wounds and scars, emotionally warming and opening, frustration, irritability, jealousy, lack of compassion, loneliness, rage, resentment, shock, spiritual engagement, stubbornness and trauma.

Chakra: 2nd (sacral), 3rd (solar plexus), 4th (heart)

History: Its common name is *immortelle*, or *everlasting*, as the flowers do not wither. It has been used for centuries in culinary dishes for its slight curry flavor. The flower heads are often used in herbal teas and in Midsummer Day bouquets as a symbol of eternal love.

Personal Experience: I use this essential oil for any skin irritation, discoloration, hyperpigmentation and scarring. For emotions, I find it grounding yet lifting my mind to be free of clutter and emotional baggage. It helps calm anger and heated emotions and infusing them with love, acceptance and peace.

Contraindications: Non-irritating.

Ho Leaf (*Cinnamomum camphora ct linalool; ct 1,8 cineole*)

Scent: Rich, warm, wood, balsamic scent with refreshing and earthy undertones

Note: Middle 6

Extraction Method: Steam Distillation

Parts Used: Leaves and twigs

Plant Description: It is a fire-resistant, evergreen tree that can grow up to 50-150 feet and has a wide trunk. It has smooth braches with alternating, dark green, glossy leaves, that when crushed, disperse its camphor scent. It has tiny, cream-colored flowers that produce many round, pea-sized purple-black berries. The camphor tree can grow in full sun or partial shade, with fertile, sandy, alkaline soil. It grows poorly in wet soils. Mature trees can be drought tolerant as well as survive freezes. Their root systems can multiply quickly especially as they get older, which sometimes can smother surrounding areas. It is a member of the Lauraceae family. This tree produces two essential oils, ho leaf from the leaves and camphor from the wood.

Properties: Analgesic, antibacterial, anti-inflammatory, antiseptic, antiviral, aphrodisiac, expectorant, febrifuge, mucolytic, rubefacient and sedative yet stimulating.

Chemistry: Ketones (fenchone, thujone, piperitone); Oxides (1,8 cineole); Monoterpinol (borneol); Diterpenes (camphorene); Monoterpenes (pinene, camphene, limonene, terpinene); Sesquiterpenes (linalool, terpineolene); and Phenols (safrole).

Main Body Systems: Immune, respiratory, structural

Physical: Bronchitis, colds, cough, diabetes, fever, immune support, intestinal discomfort, lymphatic congestion, muscles aches and pains, joint issues, neuralgia, relaxation, rheumatoid arthritis, shingles and skin conditioner.

Mental: Anxiety, assertive, clarity, confusion, courage, depression, fatigue, focus, fortitude, grounding, hysteria, mental balance, nervousness and stress.

Emotional: Anger, apathy, disconnected, emotional strength during trying times, fear, feel defeated, grief, inner peace, irritability, panic, safe and secure, spiritual connection and warms the heart.

Chakra: 2nd (sacral), 4th (heart), 5th (throat)

History: There has been confusion in the name of Ravintsara, Ravensare, Ho Leaf and Camphor, due to a mis-translation from the Malagasian language. In their country, they call *Cinnamomum camphora,* ravintsara. Although there are similarities in the oil benefits, they are unrelated species. This is why reviewing the botanical name and source is important before employing this oil, to ensure you have what you need to accomplish your purpose. It is more commonly used in recent times as a substitute for the endangered rosewood, and used in perfumes and skin care.

Personal Experience: I use this essential oil to open respiration, boost immunity and combat muscle aches and tension. Emotionally, it helps me decongest stuck emotions, open my mind to clearer thinking and move forward with confidence and certainty.

Contraindications: Avoid during pregnancy, with epilepsy and asthmatics.

 # Hyssop *(Hyssopus officinalis)*

Scent: Sweet-earth, warm, green with floral and camphor-like undertones

Note: Middle 6-7 (1 drop can go a long way and packs a powerful punch; use sparingly)

Extraction Method: Steam Distillation

Parts Used: Leaves

Plant Description: It is an evergreen perennial shrub that can grow up to two feet. It has woody stems with small, slender leaves, similar to rosemary (not as hard) and lavender, and produces stalk-like clusters of small purplish-blue flowers. It prefers full sun exposure, but can tolerate some shade, in well-drained, sandy soil. It is drought tolerant. It is a member of the Labiatae family.

Properties: Antibacterial, antifungal, antispasmodic, antiviral, carminative, cicatrisant, diaphoretic, expectorant, febrifuge, sedative yet stimulating (circulation, digestion) and sudorific.

Chemistry: Ketones (isopinocamphone, pinocamphone, thujone); Monoterpenes (pinene, limonene, ocimene, sabinene, camphene); Sesquiterpenes (germacrene, caryophyllene); Sesquiterpenols (nerolidol, elemol); Monoterpinols; Esters; and Oxides (1,8 cineole).

Main Body Systems: Digestive, respiratory, structural

Physical: Analgesic, arthritis, asthma, candida, digestive aid, gout, liver and gall bladder support, menopause issues, PMS discomfort, respiratory concerns, toothaches and urinary concerns.

Mental: Anxiety, blood pressure regulation, cleanses the aura, concentration, creativity, fatigue, focus, insomnia, intuition, mental sluggishness and stamina, positive thinking, PTSD, release emotional pain, restless and worry.

Emotional: Anger, bruised ego, defensive, emotional recovery from trauma, fear, feel bogged down, grief, guilt, hot- temper, irritated, lashing out, opinionated, rage, sensitive, spiritual growth and suffocated.

Chakra: 1st (root), 4th (heart), 6th (third eye), 7th (crown)

History: Historically used by herbalists for pulmonary issues and as a carminative. Romans used to fight against the plague, as a disinfectant. Spiritually it was said to purify and "forgive sins". It is an old English country remedy for cuts and wounds suffered from working in the fields. It is used in the manufacture of the liquors Absinthe, Chartreuse and Benedictine.

Personal Experience: I use this essential oil to help promote a restful sleep, calm nerves, joint pain and digestive upset. Mentally I like it to inspire clear and positive thinking.

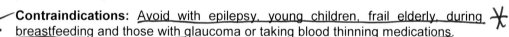

Contraindications: <u>Avoid with epilepsy, young children, frail elderly, during breastfeeding and those with glaucoma or taking blood thinning medications.</u>

Inula *(Inula graveolens, helenium)*

Scent: Sweet, herbaceous, refreshing, mint-like with sweet, stimulating undertones

Note: Middle-base 7-8

Extraction Method: Steam Distillation

Parts Used: Flowers

Plant Description: It is an herbaceous perennial plant that can grow up to two feet high. It has green, mini blade-like leaves with yellow daisy-like flowers that has numerous slender petals like sunrays. It prefers moist but well-drained, non-clay soils in warm temperatures. It is a member of the Compositae family.

115

Properties: Analgesic, anti-asthmatic antibacterial, antifungal, anti-inflammatory, antiparasitic, decongestant, diuretic, expectorant, hepatoprotective, immune stimulant, mucolytic, nervine and stomachic.

Chemistry: Oxides (1,8 cineole); Esters (bornyl acetate); Monoterpenols (borneol); Sesquiterpenols (elemol, cadinol); Monoterpenes (limonene, cymene, pinene, camphene); Sesquiterpenes (caryophyllene); and Ketones. The chemical component strength varies greatly depending on harvesting region.

Main Body Systems: Immune, nervous, respiratory

Physical: Adrenal fatigue, balances nervous system, circulation, digestive and intestinal tonic, ear, nose and throat ailments, gall bladder support, hormone balance, laryngitis, lymph drainage, muscle tension, respiratory concerns (bronchitis, dry coughs, lungs, sinuses) and shingles.

Mental: Anxiety, concentration, confusion, focus, lethargy, mental stagnation, nervousness, overwhelmed by situations, performance, productivity, speaking up for self, stamina, and stimulates the mind.

Emotional: Buried anger, deep emotional wounds, emotional cleansing, helps one cope with deep emotional issues, grief, guilt, mental instability, numb emotions, stuckness and warms the heart.

Chakra: 2nd (sacral), 4th (heart), 5th (throat), 7th (crown)

History: The name was derived from the Romans who myth says that an inula plant grew at the place where Helen of Troy's tears fell. In France and Switzerland, it is used as an ingredient in absinthe and vermouth. A common fixative in perfumes. Ancient remedies used it to loosen phlegm in cases of colds, bronchitis and emphysema. *Inula helenium* is commonly referred to as elecampane.

Personal Experience: I use this essential oil to enhance my immune system, fight off airborne germs and invaders, enhance respiration and combat chest, cough, sinus and lymphatic congestion. Emotionally it makes me feel like I have room to breathe, space to think and stamina to conquer any task at hand.

Contraindications: Skin sensitivity and irritant. Inula helenium (higher in phenols) has been shown to be more irritating so graveolens has been recommended more for aromatherapy.

Jasmine *(Jasminum officinale, grandiflorum, sambac)*

Scent: Floral, sweet, sensuous, heavy with mild-fruity undertones

Note: Middle 6

Extraction Method: Carbon Dioxide, Solvent Extraction

Parts Used: Flowers

Plant Description: It is an evergreen deciduous climbing shrub that can grow at a fast rate up to 32 feet height. It has vibrant green leaves with star-like white, aromatic flowers. It prefers moist, well-drained, acid soil in semi-shade to no shade. It can grow in sunlight, as long as it is shielded from cold winds. It is frost sensitive. It is a member of the Oleaceae (olive) family.

Properties: Analgesic, antidepressant, anti-inflammatory, antiparasitic, antiseptic, antispasmodic, antiviral, aphrodisiac, cicatrisant, euphoric, galactagogue, sedative, styptic, sudorific and uterine tonic.

Chemistry: Esters (benzyl acetate, benzyl benzoate); Diterpenes (phytol, isophytol); Monoterpenols (linalool, geraniol); Triterpenols (squalene); and Ketones.

Main Body Systems: Glandular, hepatic, nervous

Physical: Adrenal fatigue, cold extremities, breast milk production, hot flashes, impotence, liver deficiency, muscle tension and soreness, pineal gland issues, PMS, ringworm, skin irritations and uterine issues (to tonify).

Mental: Accuracy, anxiety, concentration, confidence, creativity, depression, fainting, fatigue, focus, hormone headaches, insomnia, intuition, mood swings, nervous tension, restless dreams, stress relief and uplifting.

Emotional: Anger, apathy, cold-hearted, enable ability to receive without feeling guilty, feeling vulnerable, frigidity, hysteria, irritability, post-partum depression, paranoia, restores emotional strength, self-esteem, spiritual purification and warms the heart.

Chakra: 1st (root), 2nd (sacral), 3rd (solar plexus), 4th (heart), 6th (third eye)

History: In India it is known as the Queen of the Night, and was used in ceremonial events and as offerings to the temples for spiritual purification. Chinese text describe jasmine as far back as 3rd century CE. Louis XIV was said to have slept in jasmine scented sheets. Cleopatra scented the sails of her ship to attract men. Commonly used in European gardens, and to make love sachets and incense. It is a nocturnal fragrance so flowers must be picked before daylight. Great as a perfume especially when mixed with other floral and citrus oil. Herbally, it has been scientifically noted for its use in dermatology as either an antiseptic or anti-inflammatory. All jasmines have an affinity for breast concerns, however, the sambac species is slightly more prominent for this.

Personal Experience: I use this essential oil in many of my perfumes, for skin irritations and hormone imbalances. Emotionally, I like it to relieve depression, anxiety, PTSD and to feel like I have control in my life.

Contraindications: Use caution during pregnancy. Those with allergies to the plant species.

Juniper

There are numerous types of juniper trees which belong to the *Juniperus* genus in the Cupressaceae (cypress) family. Many of the common names actually include "cedar", although true cedars belong to the *Cedrus* (cedar) genus. I will focus on two in particular that are most commonly used in aromatherapy, *Juniperus communis,* or common juniper and *Juniperus virginiana,* known as a

New World species.

√ **Juniper** *(Juniperus communis)*

Scent: Warm, herbaceous scent with floral, woody, berry and earth undertones

Note: Middle 6

Extraction Method: Steam distillation

Parts Used: Berries

Plant Description: It is a coniferous, evergreen shrub that can grow to a height of 32 feet. It has needle-like leaves and produces small blue-purple berries. The branches span out to the side like a canopy, which it hides the sunlight from whatever grown underneath. It prefers dry, acid and well-drained soil in a sunny to semi-shaded area. It can live for centuries. It is a member of the Cupressaceae family.

Properties: Antibacterial, antiseptic, antispasmodic, astringent, carminative, diaphoretic, diuretic, insecticide, rubefacient, stomachic, sudorific, tonic and vulnerary.

Chemistry: Monoterpenes (pinene, camphrene, sabinene, myrcene, terpinene, phellandrene); Esters (bornyl acetate); Monoterpenols (terpin-4-ol); Oxides (1,4 cineole); Ketones (camphor, junionone); and Sesquiterpenes (caryophyllene).

Main Body Systems: Lymphatic, structural, urinary

Physical: Arthritis, cellulite, cystitis, dandruff, digestive problems, eliminative support, flatulence, gout, joint pain, kidney concerns, lymphatic decongestant, skin detox, stimulate circulation, urinary tract issues and wound healing.

Mental: Addictions, anxiety, calms nerves, clears the mind, confidence, confusion, depression, dispels negative energy, feelings of uncleanliness, focus, mental exhaustion, restless, strengthens the brain, memory and optic nerve, willpower and worry.

Emotional: Encourages zest for life, discouraged, feel deprived and isolated, guilt, helps one face and overcome fear, *inner strength,* irritable, overwhelmed, persistence, self-acceptance, self-worth and withdrawn.

Chakra: 1st (root), 2nd (sacral), 3rd (solar plexus), 6th (third eye), 7th (crown)

History: Used to guard against the plague and contagious diseases by 15th and 16th century herbalists. Juniper and rosemary was burned in French hospitals to clear the air. Europe and Tibet used also to purify the air of contagious diseases. The berries and cones have been used to make gin. Indigenous people have traditionally used for diabetes. 17th century herbalist used for asthma, sciatica and to stimulate childbirth.

Personal Experience: I use this essential oil as a kidney tonic, for urinary issues, cellulite, edema, water retention and lymphatic congestion. Emotionally it helps to release repetitive, negative congestive thoughts and helps me move through and let go of stagnant emotions.

Contraindications: Due to possible nephrotoxic properties, it should be avoided with kidney disease. May cause respiratory allergies with those allergic to juniper pollen. Avoid during pregnancy.

Virginian (*Juniperus virginiana*)

Scent: Woodsy, earthy, deep with hints of sweet and pungent

Note: Upper base

Extraction Method: Steam Distillation

Parts Used: Wood

Plant Description: Also referred to as Pencil Cedar, Red Cedar or Silver Cedar. It is a pyramid-shaped evergreen that can grow up to 66 feet. It has long, tall trunks with firm branches, and the leaves are feather-like, flowing needles. It produces dark blue-purple berries. The wood is reddish-brown. It prefers dry, acid and well-drained soil in direct sunlight. It is drought and fire tolerant and can withstand mild winds. It is known to be one of the first trees to repopulate cleared, eroded and damaged land, and has the potential to live over 850 years. It is a member of the Cupressaceae family.

Properties: Abortifacient, antibacterial, anti-inflammatory, antiparasitic, antiseptic, antispasmodic, astringent, antiviral, diuretic, emmenagogue, expectorant, insecticide, nervine, vermifuge and vulnerary *(http://www.ncbi.nlm.nih.gov/pubmed/23297713)*.

Chemistry: Sesquiterpenes (cedrene, thujopsene, selinene); and Sesquiterpenols (cedrol, widdrol).

Main Body Systems: Nervous, structural, urinary

Physical: Acne, alopecia, arthritis, coughs, dandruff, eczema and psoriasis, joint pain, kidney and urinary support, mouth sores, oily skin, respiratory concerns, rheumatism and seborrhea.

Mental: Anxiety, authentic energy, concentration, focus, indecisive, mental strength, nervousness, protects against "people parasites" and energy zappers, self-esteem and shock.

Emotional: Anger, agitation, boundary invasion (and to establish boundaries), domineering, emotional harmony, exhaustion, feel like people are tearing you down, frustration, negativity, overshadowed, stress, tension and excessive worry that is eating away at you.

Chakra: 1st (root), 3rd (solar plexus), 6th (third eye)

History: Some junipers are given the common name "cedar," including *Juniperus virginiana*, which is widely used in cedar drawers. The reddish wood is highly prized for making cabinets, chests, fencing and other structures, especially due its strong ability to repel insects, moths, fire ants, roaches and other bugs. It is also popular in making the casing of lead pencils and is commonly used for Christmas trees. The Native American Indians historically used it for pulmonary concerns and skin issues. Other cultures used it as a deodorant, in polishes, perfumes, soaps and in insecticides.

Personal Experience: I use this essential oil to combat insects, fire ants, moths and bugs. Emotionally I have found it to help me see the positive side of a negative situation, for mental and emotional purification and to defend against invasion.

Contraindications: Can be a skin irritant if used undiluted. Avoid during pregnancy.

Lavender *(Lavandula angustifolia)*

Scent: Floral, herbaceous, clean scent with slight sweetness

Note: Middle 5

Extraction Method: Steam Distillation

Parts Used: Flowers and leaves

Plant Description: It is an evergreen shrub that can reach up to 3 feet in height. It has silvery-green bristle-like leaves, a woody stem and small lavender-purple flowers that form a small stalk-like appearance. It prefers warm temperatures and hydration in high elevations of sandy, well-drained and alkaline soil. It does not do well in the shade and is drought tolerant. It is a member of the Labiatae family.

Properties: Analgesic, antibacterial, antidepressant, anti-inflammatory, antiseptic, antispasmodic, antiviral, astringent, cardiotonic, carminative, cholagogue, digestive, febrifuge, insecticide, nervine, restorative, sedative, stomachic and vulnerary.

Chemistry: Monoterpenols (linalool, terpin-4-ol, terpineol, borneol, lavandulol); Esters (linalyl acetate, lavanulyl acetate); Monoterpenes (ocimene, limonene, pinene); Sesquiterpenes (caryophyllene, farnesene); Aldehydes (geranial, neral); Oxides (1,8 cineole); Coumarins; and ketones (octanone).

Main Body Systems: Glandular, nervous, structural

Physical: Air deodorizer, burns, circulation, digestion, hair loss, IBS, insect bites, joint and muscle pain, lymphatic congestion, muscle soreness, nausea, nerve pain, skin issues (acne, scars, eczema, psoriasis, rash) and toothache.

Mental: Anxiety, calm nerves, compulsion, cranky babies, frustration, headaches, insomnia, meditation, mental exhaustion, moodiness, nervous tension, PMS, rational thoughts, stress, tremors and worry.

Emotional: Acceptance, anger, balanced emotional state, betrayal, brings mind and body into harmony, conflicting emotions, fear, forgiveness, grief, inflexible feelings, inner peace and connection, irritability, panic-stricken, rejection, see the beauty in people and self, self-love, self-worth and shock.

Chakra: Balances higher and lower chakras to bring into harmony and balance.

History: Romans would use in bath water as fragrance. During the Bubonic Plague, it was burned in rooms to prevent the spread of the infection. Sachets were added to newly washed linen to repel insects and moths. It was worn around the necks of ladies wearing tight corsets to revive them after fainting. During the Middle Ages, it was considered an herb of love. Long time ancient remedy used to disinfect wounds. Several recent studies have shown lavender essential oil to enhance the quality of life in Alzheimer and Dementia patients *(http://www.ncbi.nlm.nih.gov/pubmed/17342790)*.

Personal Experience: I use this essential oil for just about everything. It is my "jack of all trades" oil that I use for just about every physical, mental and emotional issue.

Contraindications: Non-irritating.

✓Ledum *(Ledum groendlandicum)*   NO Internal

Scent: Warm, sharp, herbaceous scent with a slight spicy, medicinal undertone

Note: Middle

Extraction Method: Steam distillation

Parts Used: Flowers and leaves

Plant Description: It is an evergreen shrub that can reach heights of five feet. It has slender, light-green leaves with clusters of white, star-like flowers that form a ball-like appearance. It prefers moist, acid soil in full to semi-shaded areas. It is a member of the Ericaceae family.

Properties: Analgesic, antibacterial, antifungal, anti-inflammatory, antiviral, cholagogue, depurative, decongestant, diuretic, febrifuge, hepatic, insecticide, stomachic and vermifuge.

Chemistry: Monoterpenes (limonene, menthatriene, pinene, sabinene); Sesquiterpenols (p-menthadiene-8-o, ledol); Monoterpenols (terpineol); Aldehydes (myrtenal); Sesquiterpenes (selinene) and Esters.

Main Body Systems: Glandular, hepatic, immune

Physical: Bee stings, circulation, coughs, digestive upset, edema, immune support, insect bites, kidney drainage, liver issues, muscle pain due to lactic acid build up, nausea, prostate health, respiratory concerns, skin irritations (itching, dryness, flaking), sore throats and thyroid support.

Mental: Addictions, anxiety, compulsion, confusion, controlling and/or loss of control, headaches (in small amounts), insomnia, lethargy, mental blocks, mental sluggishness, nervousness, obsessive and restlessness.

Emotional: Anger, betrayal, bitterness, emotionally cold, emotional pain, envy, feel attacked, feel like you have been wronged by another, hardened heart, irritability, jealousy, resentment, revengeful and stuckness. *All Negative emotions*

Chakra: 1st (root), 3rd (solar plexus)

History: Also known as Greenland Moss or Labrador Tea. Native Americans used it as a "cure all". The leaves were once added to beer to make it headier and was a common substitute for tea leaves during the American Revolutionary War. They contain narcotic constituents such as ledel, and may be poisonous to animals. The leaves were placed in cupboards, with clothes and linens to repel moths, mice, lice and other insects.

Personal Experience: I love this essential oil for immune and respiratory support and to assist my body's eliminatory organs to function optimally. Emotionally, it helps bring balance when there is an invasion of "pesty" people and clears out painful thoughts.

 Contraindications: Over-use may cause headaches. Not for internal use.

 Lemon *(Citrus limonum)*

Scent: Sweet, tart, clean, fresh, citrus scent

Note: Top 2

Extraction Method: Cold Expression

Parts Used: Fruit rind

Plant Description: It is an evergreen shrub that can grow up to twenty feet high. It has medium to dark green, semi-glossy leaves with semi-round yellow fruit and small white, star-like flowers. It prefer warm climates as it is frost sensitive, in sandy, hydrated but well-drained, alkaline soil. It does not like the shade. Trees can produce up to 1500 lemons annually. It is in the Rutaceae family.

Properties: Antibacterial, antifungal, antiseptic, antiviral, astringent, carminative, diaphoretic, digestive, diuretic, febrifuge, fungicide, insecticide, rubefacient, stimulant, stomachic and vermifuge.

Chemistry: Monoterpenes (limonene, pinene, terpinene, sabinene, cymene); Aldehydes (citral, citronellal, neral, geranial); Monoterpenols (decanol, linalool); Esters (geranyl acetate, neryl acetate); Sesquiterpenes (bisabolene); Tetraterpenes (carotene); Coumarins; and Furanocoumarins.

Main Body Systems: Digestion, immune, nervous

Physical: Acid reflux, alkalizes pH, blood and lymph purifier, cellular congestion, cellulite, circulation, cold and flu, digestive aid, edema, erysipelas, high blood pressure, increases white blood cell activity, lymphatic drainage, neuro-hormonal dysregulation, respiratory concerns, urinary issues and vein health.

Mental: Alertness, clear thinking, concentration, confusion, depression, dispel sluggishness, doubt, fatigue, focus, imagination, inspiration, jet lag, mental clarity and congestion, nervousness, refresh a tired and stressed mind, rejuvenate mind, sound decision making and stimulate intellect and wisdom.

Emotional: Anger, clears inner conflict, connects head, heart and gut, emotional stuckness, encourages laughter, feel burdened, frustration, happiness, hopeful, impatience, irritability, joy, lifts spirits, optimistic, overwhelmed by responsibilities, resentment, security, spiritual awareness and trust in relationships.

Chakra: 3rd (solar plexus), 6th (third eye)

History: 17th century physicians used as a blood cleanser and carminative. The British navy gave sailors an ounce a day during sea voyages to prevent and treat scurvy and other nutrient deficiency diseases. The fruit contains significant amounts of vitamins C and A, which helps the body fight off infections. Often used in cosmetics as a skin brightener, and in hair care products as a hair lightener. It is added to many culinary dishes for flavor and as a digestive aid.

Personal Experience: I use this essential oil for many reasons, and it is in my top 10 must-haves. This bottle of sunshine boosts my immune system when I need it, relieves respiratory and chest congestion, lifts mood, puts a smile on my face, promotes creativity and imagination, focus, concentration and memory recall. Emotionally it helps decongest stuck and sluggish emotions.

Contraindications: Photosensitive.

Lemongrass *(Cymbopogon citratus, flexuosus)*

Scent: Lemon-scent, fresh, green, herbaceous with sweet undertones

Note: Middle 6-7

Extraction Method: Steam Distillation

Parts Used: Grass

Plant Description: It is an evergreen shrub that has strong, course, blade-like grass that grows up and flops over, like a water fountain. It can grow up to five feet high. It prefers dry, well-drained, acid soil in sunny climates, but can also grow in semi-shaded areas, as long as it gets more than a half days sunlight. It is a member of the Poaceae family.

Properties: Analgesic, antibacterial, antidepressant, antifungal, antiseptic, antispasmodic, antiviral, astringent, carminative, deodorant, diuretic, febrifuge, galactagogue, insecticide, nervine, stimulant and stomachic.

Chemistry: Aldehydes (geranial, neral, farnesol); Monoterpenols (geraniol, citronellol, terpineol); Sesquiterpenes (farnesol); Esters (geranyl acetate, linalyl acetate); Monoterpenes (myrcene, limonene); Sesquiterpenols (caryophyllene); Oxides; and Ketones.

Main Body Systems: Circulation (cephalic), immune, lymphatic

Physical: Air purifier and deodorizer, colds and flu, digestive aid, headache, herpes, immune support, indigestion, intestinal parasites, lymphatic congestion, muscle stiffness, neuralgia, nutrient absorption, respiratory concerns, shingles, spleen health, sore throats, thymus gland support and tones muscles and connective tissues.

Mental: Alertness, brain fog, communication, concentration, confidence, creativity, depression, energizing, focus, jet lag, inspiration, lifts mood, mental clarity, mental fatigue, mood swings, negativity, nervousness, vitality and worry.

Emotional: Emotional congestion, fear, flexible to change, fright, frustration, guilt, healed emotions, hopeful, hypersensitivity, inner strength, inspires personal power, joy, judgmental, let go of past hurt, self-esteem, self-love and weakness.

Chakra: 3rd (solar plexus), 4th (heart), 6th (third eye)

History: Ayurveda medicine uses for coughs and nasal congestion. Chinese medicine uses for headaches, stomach-aches and rheumatic pains. In East India and Sri Lanka it is referred to as the "fever tea" and also employed for PMS, diarrhea and stomach issues. It is often used by many cultures in culinary dishes for its taste and preservative properties. It is a close relative to the citronella plant and known to repel insects and bugs. It is also commonly employed in perfumes.

Personal Experience: I use this essential oil in my hand sanitizer as a disinfectant and to boost immunity, for lymphatic decongestant and as a digestive aid. Emotionally it clears my head, promotes vibrant, positive and creative thinking and enables more pure visualization.

Contraindications: May cause skin irritation to those with sensitive skin.

Lime *(Citrus medica)*

Scent: Fruity, sweet, uplifting, tangy

Note: Top 1-2

Extraction Process: Cold Expression

Parts Used: Fruit rind or juice

Plant Description: It is an evergreen, coniferous tree that can grow to heights of 18 feet. It has vibrant green, semi-glossy leaves, small white or yellow flowers with round green fruits. The trunk is strong and often used as firewood. It prefers sandy, hydrated but well-drained soil in warm, sunny climates, as it does not like the shade. It is drought tolerant and frost sensitive. It is a member of the Rutaceae family.

Properties: Antiviral, antibacterial, antiscorbutic, antiseptic, astringent, deodorant, disinfectant, diuretic, febrifuge, insecticide, restorative, stomachic, tonic and vermifuge.

Chemistry: Monoterpenes (limonene, pinene, sabinene, myrcene); Aldehydes (citral); Monoterpenols (linalool, terpineol); Esters (linalyl acetate); Sesquiterpenes (bisabolene); Furanocoumarins (bergaptene); and Ketones (fenchone).

Main Body Systems: Digestive, immune, nervous

Physical: Alkalizes pH, alopecia, anemia, brittle hair and nails, cold and flu, cellulite, edema, fever, high blood pressure, increases white blood cell activity, joint pain, lymph stagnation, overproduction of sebum (acne, cyst, oily skin), respiratory concerns, sore throat, urinary issues and viral concerns.

Mental: Anxiety, awareness, clarity, combats fatigue, cognitive support, concentration, confidence, confusion, depression, focus, headaches, mental clutter, nervous tension, rejuvenates mind and spirit, stress and worry.

Emotional: Adjust to new changes and transitions (career, location, life), anger, balance, compassion, distress, emotional fatigue, feel supported, harmony, hide feelings, inner strength, irritability, secretive, self-esteem, self-love, shy and timid.

Chakra: 3rd (solar plexus), 4th (heart), 6th (third eye)

History: It is popular in culinary dishes and alcoholic beverages as a garnish and flavor enhancer. Many places uses the dehydrated peel in cattle feed. Commonly added in household cleaners as it disinfects and cleans metal and glass with no streaks. Known for its high content of vitamin C and calcium. In India, it is used to dispel negative energy.

Personal Experience: I use this essential oil for pH balancing, lymphatic and digestive support and to help with joint pain. Emotionally it helps me adapt during times of transitions and change, keep an open mind, be optimistic and flexible.

Contraindications: Photosensitive.

Litsea cubeba – see May Chang

Mandarin, Orange *(Citrus reticulata)* – see Orange

✓**Marjoram** *(Origanum marjorana);* Spanish Marjoram *(Thymus mastichina)*

Scent: Pungent, hot, earthy and spicy with slight camphoraceous undertones

Note: Middle 5-6

Extraction Method: Steam Distillation

Parts Used: Flowers and leaves

Plant Description: It is a bushy, evergreen perennial shrub that can grow to heights of two feet tall. It has soft, fuzzy silvery-green leaves that grow very close together with knot-like white or pink flowers. It prefers sandy, hydrated but well-drained, calcium-rich soil in warm, sunny climates but does well in shaded areas as well. It has a shallow root system and is frost sensitive. It is a member of the Labiatae family.

Properties: Analgesic, antibacterial, antifungal, antiseptic, antispasmodic, antiviral, aphrodisiac, carminative, diaphoretic, diuretic, expectorant, insecticide, nervine, sedative, tonic, vasodilative and vulnerary.

Chemistry: Monoterpenes (sabinene, terpinene, cymene, myrcene); Monoterpenols (linalool, terpin-4-ol, terpineol); Esters (linalyl acetate, geranyl acetate); Aldehydes (citral); Sesquiterpenes (terpinolene); and Ethers.

Main Body Systems: Digestive, nervous, structural

Physical: Bruising, digestive aid, herpes, heart palpitations, high blood pressure, increases intestinal peristalsis, joint pain, laryngitis, muscle relaxant, PMS cramps, sinus congestion, stimulates circulation, toothaches and urinary issues.

Mental: Addictions, anxiety, confusion, dizziness, hyperactivity, hysteria, insomnia, learning abilities, memory recall, mental exhaustion, migraines, obsessive, panic, post-partum depression, relaxes nervous system, restlessness and strengthens cognitive functions.

Emotional: Ability to care, anger, emotional pain, fear, feel threatened, feeling numb, freedom and liberation from constraints, frightened, grief, heightens intuition, irritability, joy, loneliness, oppressed, promotes peace, restores enthusiasm, sadness, self-love, trauma and warms the heart.

Chakra: 3rd (solar plexus), 4th (heart), 6th (third eye)

History: In Greek, it translates to "joy of the mountains". Myths say that Aphrodite, goddess of love, beauty and fertility, first cultivated the plant. Greeks wore wreaths of marjoram as wedding flowers to bestow a long and prosperous life. It was planted on graves by loved ones of the deceased to ensure they would rest in peace. It's commonly added to culinary dishes for its antioxidants properties which help it preserve foods.

Personal Experience: I use this essential oil for nerve pain, headaches, IBS and PMS cramps, muscle spasms and to calm nerves to promote a restful sleep. Emotionally, it helps with emotional pain and trauma, giving me room to breathe (like from the top of a mountain) and promoting self-love.

Contraindications: Over use may contribute to low blood sugar and decreased libido.

May Chang *(Litsea cubeba)*

Scent: Lemony, sweet with green, herbaceous undertones

Note: Middle 4-5

Extraction Process: Steam Distillation

Parts Used: Fruit

Plant Description: It is a deciduous evergreen tree that can grow up to thirty feet tall. It has bright green lemon-scented leaves, clusters white flowers with yellow stamens (looks like popcorn from a distance) on stalks and small, round berries. It prefers sandy, moist and acidic soil in full sunlight, but does well in partial shade as well. It is a member of the Lauraceae family.

Properties: Analgesic, antibacterial, anti-inflammatory, anti-depressant, antifungal, antiseptic, antispasmodic, antiviral, carminative, diuretic, expectorant, febrifuge, galactagogue, hypotensive, insecticide, tonic and vulnerary.

Chemistry: Aldehydes (citral, neral, geranial); Monoterpenols (geraniol, linalool, citronellol); Esters (linalyl acetate); Sesquiterpenes (cadinene); Monoterpenes (limonene, sabinene); and Oxides (cineole).

Main Body Systems: Digestive, glandular, nervous

Physical: Athlete's foot, arthritis, calms the heart, chills associated with cold and flu, digestive aid, excess heat and perspiration, pain and swelling, regulates body temperature, relaxes nerves, restful sleep,

Mental: Anxiety, communication, confidence, depression, dizziness, energizing, fatigue, headache, hysteria, insomnia, invigorates mood, memory weakness, mental stimulant, relaxes nerves, stress and uplifting.

Emotional: Abandonment issues, adapt to change, compassion, emotional clarity, feel isolated, frozen with emotion, help one work through emotional conflict, self-doubt, self-worth and warms cold emotions.

Chakra: 2nd (sacral), 3rd (solar plexus), 4th (heart), 6th (third eye)

History: It is commonly referred to by its botanical name, but in China, it is referred to as May Chang. It has been a part of Asian and Indian herbal medicine, cuisines, perfumes and soaps for centuries. It has been used for travel sickness and to dispel internal wind (gas) and coldness.

Personal Experience: I use this essential oil for muscle and joint pain, soreness and swelling, to calm nerves, invigorate the mind and promote articulation. Emotionally, it has been helpful in warming cold emotions and balancing emotional struggles.

Contraindications: Photosensitive.

Melissa *(Melissa officinalis)* ✓

Scent: Lemon, honey-like, semi-sweet, green scent with hints of balsamic undertones

Note: Middle 5-6

Extraction Method: Steam Distillation

Parts Used: Flowers and leaves

Plant Description: It is a perennial plant that can grow up to two feet tall. It has green leaves with an embossed texture and serrated edges. The flowers are white and pink. It prefers sandy, well-drained, acid soil in semi-shaded to no shade areas. It is frost and drought tolerate. It is a member of the Labiatae family.

Properties: Analgesic, antibacterial, antidepressant, anti-inflammatory, antispasmodic, antiviral (strong), carminative, diaphoretic, emmenagogue, febrifuge, hypotensive, insecticide, nervine, sedative and stomachic.

Chemistry: Aldehydes (geranial, neral, citronellal); Sesquiterpenes (caryophyllene); Esters (geranyl acetate, neryl acetate); and Phenols (carvacrol, eugenol).

Main Body Systems: Circulation (cardiovascular), immune, glandular

Physical: Asthma, bronchitis, calm hyperactive thyroid, chronic fatigue, cold sores, Epstein-barr, facial tics, GI spasms, gout, heart palpitations, herpes, hysteria, hypertension, indigestion, nausea, neuropathy pain, PMS, urinary issues and vertigo.

Mental: Addictions (smoking, drinking, anorexia, OCD), anxiety, confusion, creativity, dementia, depression, exhaustion, headache, hysteria, insomnia, mental blocks, migraine, nervous tension, panic attacks and strengthens brain function.

Emotional: Abandonment, acceptance, anger, comforts the heart, fear of confrontation, feel defeated and attacked, grief, guilt, inner contentment, low self-esteem, irritability, lifts spirits, rejection, sadness, shock and trauma.

Chakra: 1st (root), 3rd (solar plexus), 4th (heart), 5th (throat), 6th (throat)

History: 16th century physicians revered as an "elixir of life" and used it as an antidepressant and a memory enhancer. German studies found this oil to be effective for viruses such as herpes, smallpox, mumps and flu. The plant was often times rubbed on skin to repel mosquitoes and insects. Dr. Florian Birkmayer uses it to calm and decrease stress, relieve anxiety and promote inner contentment.

Personal Experience: I use this essential oil to combat virus issues, nerve pain, anxiety and to replenish after times of exhaustion and over-giving. Emotionally it helps me stick to my boundaries without invasion and to stand in my own power.

Contraindications: Photosensitive.

Monarda *(Monarda fistulosa)*

Scent: Lemony, herbaceous with floral, pungent and camphoraceous undertones

Note: Middle 6

Extraction Method: Steam distillation

Parts Used: Flowers and leaves

Plant Description: It is a perennial plant that can grow up to five feet high. It has light to dark green, coarse surfaced, heart-shaped leaves with slender, pointy petals of lavender, pink, red and white flowers that look like a firework. It prefers semi-dry, well-drained, alkaline soil in full sun to partial shade, but not complete shade. Can tolerate some drought but doesn't thrive when over-watered. It is a member of the Labiatae family.

Properties: Analgesic, antibacterial, anti-inflammatory, antiseptic, antiviral, carminative, diaphoretic, diuretic, emmenagogue, expectorant, febrifuge, nervine, sedative and stimulant.

Chemistry: Phenols (thymol, carvacrol, hydrothymoquinone); Monoterpenes (cymene, limonene, pinene); Monoterpenols (linalool, geraniol, nerol); Esters; and Aldehyde (geranial, aliphatic aldehyde).

Main Body Systems: Hepatic, nervous, respiratory

Physical: Chilliness, colic, enhances circulation, gall bladder support, hot flashes, heated liver issues, hyperacidity, IBS, indigestion, muscle and nerve pain, night sweats, respiratory congestion, seborrhea, skin issues (acne, eczema, irritation, wounds), sore throat and urinary concerns.

Mental: Brain circulation, calms nerves, clarity, communication, confidence, dementia, fatigue, headache, insomnia, inspiration, memory recall, mental clarity, restless sleep, restores mind and worry excessively.

Emotional: cold emotions, connected to true self, disappointment, discontent, emotional strength, fear something bad will happen, harmonizes spirit, ignite passion, joy, personal transformation, rejection, sadness, self-esteem, self-forgiveness, self-worth, trust self and warm hearted.

Chakra: 3rd (solar plexus), 4th (heart), 5th (throat)

History: In Europe, it is referred to it as "golden melissa" or "Indian nettle." It is commonly called bee balm, wild bergamot or horsemint. It was named by Linnaeus to honor a Spanish physician-botanist and author, Nicolas Monardes (1493-1588), who wrote about many New World plants. North American Indians developed its medicinal use, and commonly employed it to alleviate stomach and bronchial ailments. It has been described by ancient healers as a "sweet leaf" for its fragrance and taste. It was used as a tea substitute during the Boston Tea Party boycott.

Personal Experience: I use this essential oil to calm nerves, balance my heart rhythm when stressed, combat respiratory congestion and to cool fevers and excessive body heat. Emotionally it helps me connect to my inner strength and purpose. It keeps me true to myself, and not give in to negative emotions.

Contraindications: Non-irritating.

✓ Myrrh *(Commiphora myrrha)*

Scent: Clean, fresh, brown, warm scent with an ever-so slight hint of a spice undertone

Note: Base 8 (1 drop can "mute" a blend)

Extraction Method: Steam distillation or carbon dioxide

Parts Used: Resin

Plant Description: It is a large shrub that can grow up to ten feet high. It has a gnarly, knotted trunk and branches with spike-like bark that exudes a sap, in which the dried resin is used to make the essential oil. The small scanty, slender, glossy green leaves spread out among the branches to somewhat form a canopy. It prefers sandy, dry soil in dry climates. It is a member of the Burseraceae family.

Properties: Analgesic, antibacterial, antifungal, anti-inflammatory, antiseptic, antiviral, astringent, carminative, digestive, emmenagogue, expectorant, mucilage, pulmonary stimulant, sedative, tonic and vulnerary.

Chemistry: Sesquiterpenes (lindestrene, elemene, copaene); Furanoids (methoxyfurogermacrene, furoendesmadiene); Ketones (curzenone); Monoterpenes (ocimene, pinene, cadinene); Triterpenes (amyrin); Aldehydes (cuminaldehyde); Carboxylic Acids; and Phenols.

Main Body Systems: Immune, respiratory, structural

Physical: Aging process, bleeding gums, cold sores, constipation and diarrhea, debility, degeneration, dry and catarrh cough, increases white blood cell activity, indigestion, laryngitis, PMS cramps, respiratory congestion, skin repair (scars, wounds), sore throat and wasting conditions.

Mental: Anxiety, communication, creative blocks, determination, express thoughts, inspires purpose, mediation, mental clarity, motivation, mutism, negativity, nervous tension, overthinking, over-worrying, speech issues and strengthens the mind.

Emotional: Anger, coldness, emotional stability and weakness, frustration, grief and loss, grounding, helps release past burdens to enable one to move forward, inner stillness, purification, rejection, repression, shock, speak up for self, spiritual awareness and connection, tranquil feelings and trauma.

Chakra: 1st (root), 2nd (sacral), 5th (throat), 7th (crown)

History: It was one of the gifts of the magi and more prized than gold. Egyptians used as an incense during ceremonies, as part of the embalming and mummification process as well as burned it at funerals to honor the deceased. Greeks used to treat battle wounds. A common ingredient of toothpowders and employed in cosmetics for its preservative and anti-aging benefits. It is the longest essential oil to distill.

Personal Experience: I use this essential oil for respiratory concerns, sore throat, skin irritations and wounds, thyroid support and as a base in perfumes. Emotionally it helps me articulate and speak up for myself and work through emotional trauma so I can stay grounded and move forward.

Contraindications: Non-irritating.

✓ Myrtle *(Myrtus communis)*

Scent: Herbaceous, green with woody, balsamic, citrusy and spicy undertones

Note: Middle 5-6

Extraction Method: Steam distillation

Parts Used: Leaves

Plant Description: It is an evergreen tree that can grow up to 16-22 feet high. It has dark green, smooth, glossy leaves with small white, star-like flowers with stamens that give the appearance of a sparkler and produce a blue berry that has a spicy aroma and flavor. It prefers sandy, hydrated but well-drained soil in full to partial sunlight, but not full shade. It is frost sensitive and needs to be protected from cold winds. It is a member of the Myrtaceae family.

Properties: Analgesic, antibacterial, antiparasitic, antiseptic, antispasmodic, antiviral, astringent, carminative, decongestant, expectorant, homeostatic, immune stimulant, sedative, uterine tonic and vulnerary.

Chemistry: Oxides (1,8 cineole); Monoterpenes (pinene, limonene); Esters (myrtenyl acetate, geranyl acetate); Monoterpenols (linalool, terpineol, myrtenol); Aldehydes (myrtenal); Phenols (myrtenol); Furanoids; and Lactones.

Main Body Systems: Digestive, glandular, respiratory

Physical: Acne, cold and flu, diarrhea, digestive aid, dry cough, earache, edema, gingivitis and gum health, hemorrhoids, respiratory concerns and strength, rheumatism, liver and gall bladder congestion, sinus congestion, thyroid issues and urinary issues.

Mental: Anxiety, comprehension, distracted easily, fatigue, insomnia, intuition, know right from wrong, memory, mental sluggishness, nervousness, irrational behavior, secretive (hide details) and verbal expression.

Emotional: Anger, beauty, blame, conflicting emotions, content, despair, discouragement, fear, harmony, irritability, let go of past emotional wounds, loneliness, peace, repression, sadness, self-love, speaking up for self without guilt, self-worth, victory, weepiness and withdrawn.

Chakra: 4th (heart), 5th (throat)

History: There are two main types of myrtle – green and red. Green myrtle is most common in aromatherapy. Egyptians used for facial tics. Romans and several other cultures used in bridal bouquets as it was a symbol of love and honor. Hippocrates, Pliny and others used medicinally for respiratory and urinary concerns. India considered it to be useful for cerebral issues. Traditional Chinese Medicine used it for sinus infections. Popular in many ancient culinary dishes and wine to add a spicy flavor. Commonly used in soaps, perfumes and skin care products.

Personal Experience: I use this essential oil for various respiratory concerns, thyroid and adrenal support. The red myrtle has helped to calm an over-excited thyroid. And the green myrtle has helped support and nourish a sluggish thyroid. Emotionally it helps me balance demands and responsibilities without feeling overwhelmed or guilty for taking time to replenish myself.

Contraindications: Over-exposure may lower blood sugar. Do not use with young children and those in liver distress.

✓ **Neroli** *(Citrus aurantium var. amara)*

Scent: Fresh, floral, citrusy orange blossom scent with warm fragrant tones

Note: Middle 6

Extraction Method: Steam Distillation

Parts Used: Flowers and leaves

Plant Description: It is an evergreen tree that can grow up to 30 feet high. It has small white, fragrant flowers that are clustered together, a bitter orange fruit and glossy two-tone leaves, dark green on top and light green on the bottom. It thrives best in warm climates, full sun in sandy, well-drained soil. It is frost sensitive. It is a member of the Rutaceae family. This tree produces three different essential oils - bitter orange from the fruit rind, petitgrain from the leaves and neroli oil from the blossoms.

Properties: Antibacterial, antispasmodic, antiseptic, aphrodisiac, carminative, deodorant, digestive, emmenagogue, euphoric, expectorant, febrifuge, hypnotic, nervine, sedative, stomachic and vermifuge.

Chemistry: Esters (linalyl acetate, geranyl acetate, neryl acetate); Monoterpenols (linalool, geraniol, terpineol); Monoterpenes (myrcene, ocimene, cymene); Aldehydes; Phenols; and Furanocoumarins.

Main Body Systems: Glandular, nervous, structural

Physical: Acne, adrenal support, arthritis, bronchitis, cholesterol, cold and flu (runny nose), constipation, heart health, intestinal sluggishness, menopausal and PMS issues, respiratory concerns, skin support (irritations, sensitive, mature skin) and weight management.

Mental: Addiction, antidepressant, concentration, confidence, confusion, creativity, depression (general and post-partum), hysteria, insomnia, mental stability and strength, motivation, nervousness, restlessness and worry.

Emotional: Agitation, anger, bitterness, blame, despair, disappointment, eating disorders, emotional pain and repression, grief, grounding, joy, irritability, loneliness, peace, resentment, sadness, shock, trauma and weepiness.

Chakra: 2nd (sacral), 3rd (solar plexus), 4th (heart), 6th (third eye), 7th (crown)

History: Popular in perfumes and skin care products. Widely associated with weddings and included in the bridal bouquets in many cultures as a symbol of innocence and purity. Crete brides and grooms were sprinkled with orange blossom water. It was also used in Madrid as a seductive perfume by prostitutes. It is referenced to Nerola, Italy, where a 17th century princess made neroli oil a highly sought after fragrance.

Personal Experience: I use this essential oil in many perfumes, to balance mood, depression, anxiety, grief and conflicting emotions. It is wonderful in skin care such as a toner or moisturizer as I've found it to strengthen and tone skin.

Contraindications: Avoid during pregnancy as it is a uterine stimulant.

✓ **Niaouli** *(Melaleuca viridiflora, quinquinervia)*

Scent: Camphor-like, fresh, clean with a touch of sweet and floral undertones

Note: Middle 5-6

Extraction Method: Steam Distillation

Parts Used: Leaves

Plant Description: It is a sprawling tree with gnarly branches and dull green leaves. It can grow up to an average of 40 feet high, but some grow taller. Its furry, bristle-like pink, red and yellow flowers have bulbs on the ends, green berries in the middle and are arranged in clusters on a stalk (resembling a bottle brush). It prefers very moist, clay soil in warm climates. It is a member of the Myrtaceae family.

Properties: Analgesic, antibacterial, anti-catarrhal, antifungal, anti-inflammatory, antiseptic, antispasmodic, antiviral, cicatrisant, diaphoretic, expectorant, febrifuge, insecticide, stimulant, vermifuge and vulnerary.

Chemistry: Oxides (1,8 cineole); Monoterpenes (pinene, limonene); Sesquiterpenols (viridiflorol, nerolidol); Monoterpenols (terpineol); Sesquiterpenes (caryophyllene); and Aldehydes.

Main Body Systems: Immune, respiratory, structural

Physical: Arthritis, bronchitis, chest congestion, colds, cough (wet), cystitis, insect bites, intestinal parasites, muscle aches, poor circulation, neuralgia, sinusitis, skin irritations (acne, burns, boils, redness, cyst), stimulates white blood cell activity, sore throat and urinary tract issues.

Mental: Anxiety, clarity, communication, concentration, depression, focus, headache, mental fatigue and sluggishness, nervousness, panic attacks, power struggle, recover and well-being after being sick, sleepiness and worry.

Emotional: Emotional repression, emotional weakness, fear, feel invaded, grief, guilt, inner contentment, let go of past hurts, lonely, lift spirits, need room to breathe to avoid suffocation, refresh the mind, sadness, self-awareness and weepiness.

Chakra: 2nd (sacral), 5th (throat)

History: The bark was used for shelter, bedding, cooking, fire and fishing gear. Traditional medicine used an infusion from the leaves for coughs, colds, congestion, headache and fever. France employed it for respiratory issues and to disinfectant medical facilities. In New Caledonia, it was credited to combating malaria. It is commonly added in toothpastes and mouthwashes as an antiseptic. The Middle East uses it for intestinal sluggishness.

Personal Experience: I use this essential oil in my skin care products to combat combination skin and acne, to boost immunity, combat muscle fatigue and enhance respiration. Emotionally it clears out stuckness and congestion to make way for positive thinking and motivation.

Contraindications: May cause skin sensitivity.

✓ Nutmeg *(Myristica fragrans)*

Scent: spicy, warm, herbaceous with camphoraceous, bitter undertones

Note: Middle 6-7

Extraction Method: Steam Distillation

Part Used: Seed

Plant Description: It is an evergreen tree that can grow up to 65 feet tall. It has dark-green shiny leaves, with strong scented, small, waxy ivory or yellow flowers. The fruit is about the size of a lemon, and as it matures, it splits in two, exposing the pulp surrounding the dark brown-purple seed (nutmeg), which is covered by a reddish-coral web-like membrane (mace). It prefers moist, well-hydrated soil in warm, sunny climates. It does not like cold weather. It is a member of the Myristicaceae family.

Properties: Analgesic, antibacterial, antifungal, anti-inflammatory, antispasmodic, antiviral, antiseptic, aphrodisiac, carminative, digestive, emmenagogue, expectorant, febrifuge and stimulant.

Chemistry: Monoterpenes (sabinene, pinene, limonene, myrcene); Ethers (myristicin, elemicin); Phenols (terpin-4-ol); Oxides (1,8 cineole); Monoterpinols; and Sesquiterpenes.

Main Body Systems: Intestinal, nervous, structural

Physical: Alopecia, arthritis, boost immunity, bronchitis, coughs (dry), diarrhea, digestive aid (fats, starches), GI upset, gout, joint and muscle pain, kidney concerns, liver concerns, nausea, parasites, PMS cramps, rheumatism, sciatica, stimulate circulation, toothaches and urinary issues.

Mental: Absentminded, addiction, anxiety, creativity, enhance dreams, fainting, headaches, insomnia, invigorates the mind, general debility, dizziness, inflexible to change, mental stimulation, lifts mood, nervous fatigue, sluggish and vertigo.

Emotional: Abandonment, alone, anger, bitterness, cold-hearted, despair, emotionally exhausted, fear, feel confined, frigidity, grief, hides true feelings, inner conflict, invasion of boundaries, resentment, sorrow and warms the heart.

Chakra: 1st (root), 3rd (solar plexus), 6th (third eye)

History: The tree provides two spices derived from its fruit - nutmeg (tree's fruit seeds) and mace (dried, fleshy seed coating). Nutmeg is commonly added in culinary dishes, beverages and desserts. Egyptians used it in the embalming process. Italians used it to ward off the plague. Greeks and Romans used as a brain tonic. Ayurveda medicine employed it for headaches, fever and intestinal disorders.

Personal Experience: I use this essential oil to calm silent reflux and nourish the GI tract to help with digestive issues. Also has helped with joint and nerve pains, muscle fatigue and dry coughs. Emotionally it alleviates congested thoughts and emotions, brings a sense of comfort and adds spice to life.

Contraindications: May cause skin irritations. Over-exposure may cause over-intoxication, nausea, hallucinogenic effects and headaches. Not for ingestion.

Oakmoss (*Evernia prunastri*)

Scent: Rich, balsamic, woody, smoky, earthy with slight bitter and sweet undertones

Note: Base 9-10

Extraction Method: Solvent extraction, Steam Distillation

Part Used: Whole plant

Plant Description: It is a fruticose lichen that grows at a slow rate on top of trees (oaks, other conifer and deciduous trees), rocks and dead wood. It has a silver-green, bushy, rubbery, sponge-like appearance with forked ends. It thrives in a moisture rich environment, with sunlight and fresh air. It can adapt to extreme climates. It is a member of the Usneaceae family.

Properties: Antibacterial, antifungal, anti-inflammatory, antioxidant, anti-parasitic, antiseptic, demulcent, expectorant and vulnerary.

Chemistry: Phenols (methyl B-orcinolcarboxylate), Aldehydes (atranorin, chloratranorin, ethyl everninate, ethyl hematommate, ethyl chlorohematommate) *(http://www.ncbi.nlm.nih.gov/pubmed/19272096)*; Carboxylic Acids (evernic acid); Monoterpenes (pinene, camphene, phellandrene, limonene) *(http://www.asianjournalofchemistry.co.in/user/journal/viewarticle.aspx?ArticleID=23_5_11)*. *(Robert Tisserand, Essential Oil Safety: A Guide for Health care Professionals, 2015; Cropwatch 'Fragrant Lichen' Bibliography: [Oakmoss/Treemoss/ Cedarmoss etc.] Compiled by Cropwatch May 2009 v1.10)*

Main Body Systems: Intestinal, structural, urinary

Physical: Alopecia, balding, constipation, digestive weakness, heartburn, liver and kidney disharmony, muscle and joint support, respiratory concerns, skin irritations (itching, eczema, dryness), teeth sensitivity, sinus issues and vaginal issues.

Mental: Addictions, ambitious, anxiety, calming, confidence, controlled and controlling, dependent and co-dependent, domineering, enhance understanding, grounding, headaches, mental strain, obsessive behaviors and quiets the mind to enjoy the moment.

Emotional: Agitation, arrogant, content, emotional openness, feelings of hopelessness, frigidity, insecure, irritability, low self-esteem, opinionated, parasitic relationships, resolves past emotional wounds, sadness, self-centered and trusting issues.

Chakra: 1st (root), 2nd (sacral), 3rd (solar plexus)

History: Most popularly used as a fixative in perfumes and colognes. Baskets filled with oakmoss were found in the royal tombs of ancient Egypt. Lichens in general were used in the commercial dye trade in Scotland.

Personal Experience: I use this essential oil for digestive upset, fungal issues and weepy skin irritations. It makes a great base note in perfumes and soaps. Emotionally it is grounding, calming, stabilizing and centering.

Contraindications: Phototoxic and may cause skin sensitivities.

√ Oranges: Bitter and Sweet

Orange, Bitter *(Citrus aurantium)*

Scent: Fruity, bittersweet, invigorating scent

Note: Top 1-2

Extraction Method: Cold Expression

Part Used: Fruit rind

Plant Description: It is an evergreen tree that has a rounded top and can grow as tall as 40 feet high. The leaves are dark green on the top, with a paler green underside. It has white, star-like flowers and round orange fruit. It prefers warm, sunny climates in sandy, moist but well-drained soil. It does not do well in full shade, and is disease resistant. It is a member of the Rutaceae family.

Properties: Anti-allergenic, antibacterial, antidepressant, antioxidant, antispasmodic, antiviral, carminative, decongestant, digestive, expectorant, febrifuge, insecticide, nervine, stomachic, tonic and vulnerary.

Chemistry: Esters (linalyl acetate, geranyl acetate, neryl acetate); Monoterpenols (linalool, geraniol, terpineol); Monoterpenes (myrcene, ocimene, cymene); Aldehydes; Phenols; and Furanocoumarins.

Main Body Systems: Circulatory, immune, nervous

Physical: Acne, adrenal exhaustion, appetite stimulant and suppressant, blood purifier, cardiotonic, colds/flu, constipation, gall bladder issues, GI upset, IBS, immune support, intestinal upset, lymphatic decongestant, skin irritations and vein health.

Mental: Addictions, anxiety, boredom, confusion, creativity, depression, focus, hyperactivity, insomnia, jet lag, mental chatter, mental fatigue, mood swings, nervousness, negativity, perfectionist, PTSD, refreshes mind, stress and uplifting.

Emotional: Anger, brings emotions into balance, distress, emotional fatigue, emotionally responsible, feels neglected, harmony, heartache, humiliation, invigorating, irritability, lonely, revitalizes spirit, sadness, stubbornness, trauma and vivacious.

Chakra: 1st (root), 2nd (sacral), 4th (heart), 5th (throat), 6th (third eye)

History: Contains a high amount of Vitamin C. Very common in culinary dishes, desserts and beverages. It is also popular in weight loss products because it enhances thermogenesis. It was first introduced to Italy by the crusaders in the 11th century, where it was widely used for medicinal purposes. In Crete, the bride and groom were sprinkled with orange blossom water.

136

Personal Experience: I use this essential oil to combat food cravings, lift mood, combat colds and flu and allergies. Emotionally it helps with anxiety, nervous tension, bitterness, resentment and feeling overwhelmed.

Contraindications: Photosensitive.

✔ Orange, Sweet *(Citrus sinensis)*

Scent: Fruity, sweet, uplifting scent

Note: Top 1-2

Extraction Method: Cold Expression

Part Used: Fruit rind

Plant Description: It is an evergreen tree that can grow as tall as 30 feet high. It has dark green, glossy leaves with white, star-like flowers and round orange fruit. It prefers warm, sunny climates in sandy, moist but well-drained soil. It does not do well in full shade. It is a member of the Rutaceae family.

Properties: Antibacterial, antidepressant, antioxidant, antispasmodic, antiviral, carminative, choleretic, digestive, febrifuge, insecticide, sedative yet stimulating, tonic and vulnerary.

Chemistry: Monoterpenes (limonene); Tetraterpenes (carotene); Aldehydes (citral, decanal); Monoterpenols (carveol, linalool); Ketones (carvone); Esters; Furanoids; and Sesquiterpenes.

Main Body Systems: Circulatory, immune, nervous

Physical: Acne, adrenal exhaustion, blood purifier, colds and flu, catarrh, digestive aid, cranky babies, immune support, intestinal upset, lymphatic decongestant, scars and stretchmarks, tension, thyroid support and vein health.

Mental: Anxiety, balances the mind and body, creativity, depression, focus, hyperactivity, insomnia, inspiration, jet lag, mental chatter, mental fatigue, mood swings, nervousness, over-analytical, perfectionist, PTSD, promotes positive thinking, refreshing, shock, stress and uplifting.

Emotional: Apathy, cheerful, distress, emotional strength, emotional fatigue, happy, invigorating, loneliness, negativity, pessimistic, revitalizes spirit, sadness, see the bright side of a situation, trauma and unfolds radiance.

Chakra: 1st (root), 2nd (sacral), 3rd (solar plexus), 5th (throat), 6th (third eye)

History: Contains a high amount of Vitamin C. A hybrid between the pomelo and mandarin fruits introduced in the late 15th century. It is a common addition to culinary dishes, desserts and beverages. In France and Italy, the orange flowers are used for floral water and perfumes. South American and Dutch soldiers planted citrus trees along trade routes to prevent scurvy. Spanish travelers introduced the sweet orange into the American continent.

Personal Experience: I use this essential oil for many things. It is in my top 10. It helps boost mood, positive and creative thinking, optimistic emotions and just a well-balanced attitude. Physically, I have used for scars, acne, colds and flu, immune boosting and in my hand sanitizer.

Contraindications: Photosensitive.

✓ Oregano *(Origanum vulgare, compactum)*

Scent: Herbaceous, earthy, warm and spicy

Note: Middle 7

Extraction Method: Steam Distillation

Part Used: Leaves, flowers, bark

Plant Description: It is an herbal plant that can grow up to three feet high. It has long, rhizome-like branches that produce small silver-green, purplish leaves and clusters of small purple flowers on the ends. It prefers warm climates in acid, dry but hydrated soil in semi-shaded areas. It is a member of the Labiatae family.

Properties: Analgesic, antibacterial, antifungal, anti-infectious, antiparasitic, antiseptic, antispasmodic, antiviral, carminative, cholagogue, decongestant, diaphoretic, disinfectant, emmenagogue, expectorant, insecticide, stimulant and vermifuge.

Chemistry: Phenols (thymol, carvacrol); Monoterpenes (cymene, terpinene, myrcene); Sesquiterpenes (caryophyllene); Esters (linalyl acetate); Carboxylic Acids (rosmaric acid); Ketones; and Monoterpinols.

Main Body Systems: Immune, intestinal, structural

Physical: Ant repellent, arthritis, bone strength, boost immunity, bronchitis, candida, cold and flu, constipation, digestive aid, dry coughs, fungal concerns, h-pylori, intestinal upset, low blood pressure, lice, lymphatic stagnation, muscle aches, parasite issues, pneumonia, respiratory concerns, stimulates circulation and toothache.

Mental: Confusion, decision making, depression, headache, insomnia, mental chatter, mental fatigue, nervousness, PTSD, restlessness, self-doubt, sluggish, stimulates imagination, violent behavior and worry.

Emotional: Abused, anger, cold emotions, defensive, emotional strength, feel attacked, frustration, grief, heartache from a toxic relationship, lonely, loss of self-identity, promote feelings of being supported, sensitive, rejection, trauma, warms a wounded heart and withdrawn.

Chakra: 1st (root), 3rd (solar plexus), 4th (heart), 6th (third eye)

History: A common ingredient in culinary dishes, soaps, perfumes and herbal pillows. It has been shown to have an abundance of iron, calcium and other minerals. Egyptians and Greeks planted oregano in graveyards to instill peace. It was customary for Greeks and Romans to crown young newlyweds with oregano, a symbol of joyous love. Pliny recommended oregano poultices for spider bites.

Personal Experience: I use this essential oil to stimulate circulation (blood and lymph) and bring warmth to cold extremities. It has also been helpful to boost immunity, combat intestinal upset and skin irritations. Emotionally, it has warmed my heart during times of feeling lost and gives strength and security.

Contraindications: Skin and eye irritant. Do not use during pregnancy.

✓Orris Root (*Iris pallida*)

Scent: Floral, powdery, violet-like with fresh, dry and herbaceous undertones

Note: Base 8

Extraction Method: Steam Distillation, Carbon Dioxide

Part Used: Root

Plant Description: It is a perennial plant that can reach heights of five feet high. It has long, narrow, dark-green, blade-like leaves, large white, blue-purple vertical and folding flowers with frilly edges and rhizomes (root). It prefers warm climates in alkaline, dry soil in semi-shaded areas. It is drought tolerant. It is a member of the Iridaceae family.

Properties: Antibacterial, antioxidant, anti-inflammatory, decongestant, deodorant, depurative, diuretic, emetic, expectorant, mucolytic, nervine, purgative and vulnerary.

Chemistry: Phenol (myristic acid); and Ketones (irone, ionone).

Main Body Systems: Glandular, hepatic, respiratory

Physical: Bronchitis, colds, coughs, diabetes, dropsy, hyperpigmentation, intestinal cramping, laryngitis, liver issues (use in small amounts), pancreas support, respiratory congestion, rheumatism, sinus issues, skin irritations (mature, dry, wrinkles), spleen support, tendons and toothaches.

Mental: Argumentative, artistic, communication, concentration, confidence, courage, creativity, depression, headache, insomnia, inspire sense of humor, intuition, lethargy, mental blocks, mental power, negativity, PTSD and wise judgment.

Emotional: Anger easily, anguish, connect to inner self, discouraged, emotional balancing, emotional wounds, fear, jealous, joy, hopeless, irritable, let inner beauty shine, personal power and protection, repression, sadness, self-love, spiritual connection and weak nerves.

Chakra: 2nd (sacral), 4th (heart), 6th (third eye)

History: Iris's symbolism in many cultures including Egyptians, is associated faith, friendship, hope, love, power and majesty. Greeks and Romans used often in perfumery, and it is still used as a fixative in perfumes today. The root is popular in Moroccan cuisine and in Russian and German beverages. Orris root powder was commonly added in European laundry to add fragrance to linens.

Personal Experience: I use this essential oil in my perfumes, skin care for

139

maturing skin and liver support. Emotionally, it has helped me connect to my personal power, true self-identity and inner beauty.

Contraindications: Not for internal use.

Palmarosa *(Cymbopogon martinii, var. motia)*

Scent: Floral, mild rose-like scent with hints of sweet, earthy and green

Note: Middle 6

Extraction Method: Steam distillation

Part Used: Grass

Plant Description: It is an herbaceous grass that is in the lemongrass genus, and can grow up to nine feet tall. It has long, slender folding leaves and flowers that are blueish when they are young and red when mature. It prefers dry, well-drained soil and sunny, humid climates. It is a member of the Gramineae family.

Properties: Antibacterial, antifungal, anti-inflammatory, antiseptic, antiviral, cardiotonic, cytophylactic, deodorant, febrifuge, insecticide, nervine, relaxant, tonic and uterine tonic.

Chemistry: Monoterpnols (linalool, geraniol); Esters (geranyl acetate, geranyl formate); Monoterpenes (dipentene, limonene, myrcene); Oxides; Sesquiterpinols.

Main Body Systems: Circulatory, digestive, hepatic

Physical: Bronchitis, calms digestive issues, colds and flu, dry cough, hypothyroid, IBS, indigestion, intestinal upset, hot flashes, neuralgia, respiratory concerns, sciatica, skin (acne, hydration, sebum balance, shingles) and urinary issues.

Mental: Anxiety, clears the mind, depression, easily distracted, fatigue, headache, helps adapt to change, hysteria, irritability, mental balance, mental congestion, nervous exhaustion, obsessive thoughts and stress.

Emotional: Anger, contentment, emotional balance, emotional strength, fear, freedom to be authentic self, inner harmony, jealous, possessive, security and trust, softens a hard heart, oppression, self-esteem, self-love and care, shock and stability.

Chakra: 1st (root), 2nd (sacral), 3rd (solar plexus), 4th (heart), 6th (third eye), 7th (crown)

History: Like geranium, it is often used to dilute or replace pure rose oil to make more affordable. Ayurveda medicine uses it for nerve pains. It was a frequent ingredient in the temple incense of the ancient Egyptians. Asian medicine used for its cooling and moistening benefits to clear excess heat in the body, mind and emotions.

Personal Experience: I use this essential oil for balancing combination skin, skin irritations and digestive upset. Emotionally, it balances, nourishes and harmonizes emotions while infusing an inner strength.

Contraindications: Non-irritating.

✓ Palo Santo *(Bursera graveolens)*

Scent: Deep, rich, earthy, woody scent with slight undertones of smoky sweet

Note: Middle to base 7-8

Extraction Method: Steam Distillation

Part Used: Wood

Plant Description: It is a tree that grows to heights of 30 feet. The silver-gray bark on the trunk is smooth and doesn't peel. The leaves are vibrant green with serrated edges and shed during dry seasons. It produces small pale-yellow flowers. It grows well in sandy, well-drained soil in sunlight. It is drought tolerant. It is a member of the Burseraceae family.

Properties: Analgesic, antibacterial, anti-catarrhal, antifungal, anti-inflammatory, antioxidant, antiseptic, antispasmodic, antiviral, cardiac tonic, decongestant, diuretic, febrifuge, insecticide, sedative and sudorific.

Chemistry: Monoterpenes (limonene, carveol); Monoterpenols (terpineol, pinene); Furanoids (menthofuran); Sesquiterpenes (germacrene, muurolene); and Ketone (carvone, pugelone).

Main Body Systems: Hepatic, respiratory, structural

Physical: Acid reflux, allergies, arthritis, cold and flu, constipation, gallstones, hormone balance, indigestion, intestinal upset, kidney, liver, lymphatic congestion, neuralgia, rheumatism, skin irritations, stomachache, toothaches and urinary discomfort.

Mental: Anxiety, clear decisions, communication, contentment, depression, determination, grounding, headache, insomnia, mental confusion, mood stabilizer, negativity, nervousness, relaxes the mind, transformation clarity, willpower and worry.

Emotional: Abandonment, ability to give and receive without guilt, anger, aura cleanse, betrayal, despair, fear, grief, heartache, protects from negative surroundings, self-reflection, shock, sorrow, spiritual connection, trauma, trusting intimate relationship and unconditional love.

Chakra: Harmonizer among chakras; 1st (root), 2nd (sacral), 3rd (solar plexus), 4th (heart), 6th (third eye), 7th (crown)

History: In Spanish it translates to "saint wood" and is commonly referred to as "holy wood". The wood was historically boiled for stomachaches, rheumatism and as an expectorant. The wood was commonly used and burned as incense for purification and to soothe the spirit. In South America it was traditionally used to cleanse your house of bad energy. Palo santo has been used in Ecuadorian clinics to help regenerate ligaments and other musculoskeletal tissues.

141

Personal Experience: I use this essential oil to help me feel centered, grounded and free from negativity. It's helpful for when I feel overwhelmed, over-burdened and drained by needy, unappreciative people. Physically, I like it to strengthen respiratory and urinary issues, and calm a nervous stomach.

Contraindications: Both Peru and Ecuador have laws governing the harvesting and export of palo santo, because the wood has become endangered through over-harvesting. Non-irritating as long as it's in a fat based carrier oil.

✓ **Parsley** (*Petroselinum sativum*)

Scent: Fresh, green, vegetative with bitter, earth undertones

Note: Middle 6-7

Extraction Method: Steam Distillation

Part Used: Leaves and/or seed

Plant Description: It is an herbaceous plant that can reach a height of two feet. The leaves are vibrant green, small and feather-like with serrated edges. It produces firework-like stalks with pale yellow flowers. It prefers acid, hydrated but well-drained, sandy soil in warm, sunny temperatures. It is a member of the Umbelliferae family.

Properties: Antibacterial, antifungal, antigalactagogue, anti-inflammatory, antioxidant, antispasmodic, carminative, deodorant, diuretic, emmenagogue, expectorant, febrifuge, hepatoprotective, hypotensive, nerve tonic and stimulant.

Chemistry: Monoterpenes (menthatriene, phellandrene, pinenemyrcene, terpinolene); Ethers (myristicin, apiole); Monoterpenols (linalool, carotol); and Sesquiterpenes.

Main Body Systems: Digestive, lymphatic, urinary

Physical: Adrenal fatigue, arthritis, circulation, digestive upset, constipation, earaches, edema, high blood pressure, liver and lymphatic congestion, nausea, night sweats, urinary concerns and wet coughs.

Mental: Cleanse negative thinking, inspire creative thinking, memory, mental blocks, motivates to take action, nervous, refreshes the mind, self-confidence, sluggishness and worry.

Emotional: Anger, bitterness, cover up faults, desire to be free, fear of moving forward, feeling attacked, feel unclean, holding on to past negative situations, jealousy, open the heart up to forgiveness and resentment.

Chakra: 3rd (solar plexus), 4th (heart)

History: According to Dr. John Christopher, parsley has a specific affinity for the adrenal glands, optic nerves and brain. The French and Middle East used historically for combating lice, painful menstruation, indigestion and reduce blood sugar. During World War I, parsley tea was used by the British soldiers for kidney complications. Used worldwide in numerous culinary dishes and as a garnish.

Personal Experience: I use this essential oil for kidney and urinary issues, digestive upset, lymphatic congestion and swelling. Emotionally it has helped me de-clutter thoughts, think more clearly without interference and work through stuckness.

Contraindications: Avoid during pregnancy as it has uterine stimulant properties, and with those with serious kidney distress.

Patchouli *(Pogostemon patchouli, cablin)*

Scent: Earthy, woody, fresh, dirt-like

Note: Middle-Base 7-8

Extraction Method: Steam distillation

Part Used: Leaves

Plant Description: It is a bushy herbaceous plant that can grow up to three feet high. The leaves are pyramidal shaped with serrated edges and a pointy tip. It has small clusters of purple-ish flowers situated on a stalk-like stem. It prefers well-hydrated, rich soil in warm climates but in the shade. It is a member of the Labiatae family.

Properties: Antibacterial, antidepressant, antifungal, anti-inflammatory, antiseptic, antiviral, aphrodisiac, cicatrisant, cytophylactic, diuretic, febrifuge, insecticide, sedative and vulnerary.

Chemistry: Sesquiterpenes (bulnesene, aromadrene, guaiene, patchoulene, germacrene); Sesquiterpenols (patchoulol); Oxides (bulnesene oxide); Ketones (patchoulenone); and Monoterpenes (pinene, limonene).

Main Body Systems: Lymphatic, structural (skin), urinary

Physical: Athlete's foot, candida, cellulite, lymphatic congestions, nail fungus, parasites and skin support (irritations, redness, itching, rash, eczema, psoriasis, dryness, scars, wrinkles, fine lines).

Mental: Addictions, anxiety, depression, exhaustion, helps people connect to their faith, enhances spirituality, indecision, insomnia, mood swings, nervousness, opens the mind, positive thinking, refuels the mind and body (especially for caretakers and nurturers) and self-doubt.

Emotional: Abandonment, ability to meditate deeply, anger, betrayal, emotional stuckness and numbness, feel neglected, grounding, harmony, helps one "let go" of what's holding them back (usually past hurts and move forward, nurturing, self-worth and stagnant emotions.

Chakra: 1st (root), 2nd (sacral), 3rd (solar plexus), 4th (heart), 7th (crown)

History: Patchouli has a historical reputation of being a "hippie oil" as it was popular in the 1960's and 1970's as an incense to cover the smell of marijuana. It is commonly used in perfumes, colognes and incense as a fixative scent. During the 18th and 19th century, silk traders from China placed dried patchouli leaves with the silk cloths packed away to combat moths from laying eggs on the cloth.

143

Personal Experience: I use this essential oil to help me feel more grounded, physically, mentally, emotionally and spiritually. It helps me let go of past hurts and grudges, to confidently and comfortably move forward. It has helped promote a restful sleep, combat fungal and parasitic issues, insect bites and itchy skin.

Contraindications: Non-irritating.

Peppermint *(Mentha piperita)*

Scent: Fresh, cool, minty, sweet, invigorating scent with earthy undertones

Note: Middle 6

Extraction Method: Steam distillation

Part Used: Leaves

Plant Description: It is an herbaceous plant that can grow up to three feet tall. It has shiny, small, crinkly leaves with serrated edges, and purple flowers. It prefers partial shade with some direct sunlight, however the roots need to be covered in cool, rich and moist but well-drained soil. Its roots can spread quickly, overtaking surrounding plants, so many prefer it to be planted in pots. It is a member of the Labiatae family.

Properties: Analgesic, antibacterial, antidepressant, antigalactagogue, anti-inflammatory, antiseptic, antispasmodic, antiviral, carminative, cephalic, decongestant, deodorant, expectorant, febrifuge insecticide and stimulant.

Chemistry: Phenols (menthol); Ketones (menthone, pulegone, piperitone); Monoterpenes (limonene, pinene, ocimene); Sesquiterpenes (germacrene); Esters (methyl acetate); Oxides (1,8 cineole, piperitone oxide); Furanoids (menthofuran); Monoterpenols (terpin-4-ol, terpineol); Sesquiterpenols (viridiflorol); and Furanocoumarins.

Main Body Systems: Digestion, hepatic, immune

Physical: Breath freshener, cold and flu, dandruff, gum health, hot flashes, indigestion, liver and lymphatic congestion, morning sickness, muscle fatigue, nausea, nerve tonic, PMS cramps, sinus issues and toothaches.

Mental: Alertness, articulation, communication, courage to speak up for self, creative clarity, depression, focus, headaches, inspires "the nerve" to conquer a task, invigorating, memory, mental fatigue, nervousness, opens mind to take in new ideas, self-doubt and stress tension.

Emotional: Anger, debility, emotionally numb and lost, fear of public speaking, frustration, grief, ignites inner passion, invigorates spirit, irritability, jealousy, self-esteem, spontaneity, suppression and weakness during confrontations.

Chakra: 3rd (solar plexus), 4th (heart), 5th (throat), 6th (third eye), 7th (crown)

History: It has long been used in numerous cultures in cooking, chewing gum, tea and toothpastes. Egyptians used it for ceremonial perfumes. Greeks used mint in temple ceremonies. Roman scholar, Pliny, considered it to be the loveliest of herbs, and remarked, "The very smell of it reanimates the spirit." Ancient

144

symbol for hospitality. Medieval Europe commonly used as a room deodorizer and flea-control agent.

Personal Experience: I use this essential oil to calm excess heat in the body (fever, PMS, hot flashes), muscle pain and fatigue, digestive and IBS upset, sore or tired feet and headaches. Emotionally it opens up my mind to take in new ideas, promoted mental clarity and allows me to have emotional strength.

Contraindications: Can be over stimulating with asthmatics when over-used.

Petitgrain *(Citrus aurantium)*

Scent: Herbaceous-floral with pungent, sweet, balsamic and woody undertones

Note: Middle 5

Extraction Method: Steam Distillation

Part Used: Leaves and twigs

Plant Description: The bitter orange tree is an evergreen that can grow up to 30 feet high. It has small white, fragrant flowers that are clustered together, a bitter orange fruit and glossy two-tone leaves, dark green on top and light green on the bottom. It thrives best in warm climates, full sun in sandy, well-drained soil. It is frost sensitive. It is a member of the Rutaceae family. This tree produces three different essential oils - bitter orange from the fruit rind, petitgrain from the leaves and neroli oil from the flower blossoms.

Properties: Antibacterial, anti-depressant, anti-inflammatory, antiseptic, antispasmodic, antiviral, carminative, deodorant, nervine, sedative and tonic.

Chemistry: Esters (linalyl acetate, geranyl acetate, neryl acetate); Monoterpenols (linalool, geraniol, terpineol, nerol); Monoterpenes (myrcene, ocimene, cymene); Aldehydes; Phenols; Sesquiterpenes (nerolidol); and Furanocoumarins.

Main Body Systems: Circulatory, glandular, nervous

Physical: Acne, adrenal burnout, appetite suppressant, calms rapid heart rate, enhanced gut-brain communication, excessive sweating, indigestion, skin irritations (blemishes, oily) and spasms (intestinal, muscles, nerves).

Mental: Addictions, anxiety, calms nervous system, compulsions, depression, inspires intellect, lifts mood, nervous exhaustion, panic, positive thinking, promote a tranquil sleep, relaxation, restlessness and stress.

Emotional: Ability to release control and ask for help, anger, avoid emotions, bitterness, comforting, denial, emotionally imbalanced, fear, judgmental of others and self, resentment, self-acceptance, self-love, shock and take time to replenish spirit.

Chakra: 1st (root), 4th (heart)

History: Mostly notably used in perfumes and colognes to tie in top and middle notes. Meaning, "little" grains", as it used to be extracted from the small unripe oranges of the tree. The leaves have historically been used along with the fruit and fruit peel as a tea for digestive issues, insomnia and gout.

Personal Experience: I use this essential oil to calm nerves, anxiety, spasms (physical, mental and emotional), and to strengthen adrenals, heart circulation and mental comprehension. Emotionally, it has helped me to combat rejection and fear while confronting my emotions and accepting help.

Contraindications: Non-irritating.

Pine *(Pinus sylvestris)*

Scent: Forest, hay-like, clean, woodsy, herbaceous scent with camphoraceous undertones

Note: Middle 5

Extraction method: Steam distillation

Part Used: Needles

Plant Description: It is a resinous, fast-growing, coniferous evergreen tree that can grow as tall as 265 feet high. The tall, slender trunks have scaly, flaking bark with hardy branches that produce green needles and oval cones. It prefers well-drained, sandy, acid or alkaline soil in shaded to sunny areas. It is very tolerant of drought, freeze and environmental pollution, as well as fire-resilient. It is a member of the Pinaceae family.

Properties: Analgesic, antibacterial, anti-depressant, anti-inflammatory, antiseptic, antiviral, aphrodisiac, decongestant, deodorant, diuretic, expectorant, rubefacient, tonic and vermifuge.

Chemistry: Monoterpenes (pinene, careen, limonene, phellandrene, sylvestrene); Sesquiterpenes (caryophyllene, cardinene); Monoterpenols (borneol); Esters (bornyl acetate); Sesquiterpinols; Diterpenes; and Aldehydes.

Main Body Systems: Glandular, respiratory, urinary

Physical: Adrenal fatigue, backaches, bronchitis, cold and flu, constipation, digestive upset, dry cough, edema, gall bladder concerns, muscle aches, respiratory congestion and weakness, rheumatism, sinus, thyroid support and urinary concerns.

Mental: Anxiety, clear vision, concentration, confidence, easily adapt to change, exhaustion, flexible, general debility, hopeful, inspire creativity, memory recall, mental fatigue, mood swings, optimism, PTSD, refreshes the mind, strengthens resilience and worry.

Emotional: Betrayal, fear, grief, guilt, invigorates the spirit, not feel supported by others, resentful, resilience through chronic stress, self-blame, self-forgiveness, self-worth, shameful, shock, speaking up for self, trauma and being "under fire".

Chakra: 2nd (sacral), 3rd (solar plexus), 4th (heart), 6th (third eye)

History: Pine wood has been used for centuries to build strong buildings, masts for sailing, furniture and paper. Hippocrates recommended it often for pulmonary issues. Native Americans, Asians and Europeans have used for urinary distress, rheumatism, arthritis and it was added to bath water for fatigue, nervous exhaustion and sleeplessness. Marguerite Maury used for rheumatism and gout.

Personal Experience: I use this essential oil to nourish my adrenals, combat respiratory congestion and urinary issues. I also include in my home cleaning products to boost mood and physical support. Emotionally, it gives me strength and endurance during times of "being under fire" and emotional distress.

Contraindications: Avoid with pine tree allergies. It has been noted to avoid long-term, over-exposure with prostate cancer, elevated PSA's, kidney and liver failure. Short term diffusion should be fine.

Ravinsara/Ravensara *(Ravintsara anisata* [bark]*; aromatica* [leaves]*; madagascareinsis* [twigs]*)*

Scent: Camphoraceous, similar to eucalyptus but sweeter and softer, invigorating with herbaceous undertones.

Note: Middle 5-6

Extraction Method: Steam distillation

Part Used: Leaves, twigs and/or bark

Plant Description: Ravinsara translated into Malagasy is Ravintsara. It is an evergreen tree that can grow up to 60 feet. It has oval, glossy leaves with small pale yellow-green flowers. It prefers well-drained, sandy soil in humid, wet climates. It is a member of the Lauraceae family.

Properties: Analgesic, anti-allergenic, antibacterial, antiviral, antiseptic, anti-inflammatory, aphrodisiac, cicatrisant, decongestant, expectorant, febrifuge, immune-stimulant, nervine, tonic and vulnerary.

Chemistry: Each part of the plant produces varying chemistry. References include Dr. Bruce Berkowsky, Robert Tisserand and Kurt Schnaubelt. The Bark has much higher Ethers (90-95% estragole).

Leaves and twigs: Monoterpenes (pinene, careen, limonene, myrcene, sabinene, terpineol); Sesquiterpenes (germacrene, caryophyllene, isoledene); Monoterpenols (linalool); Ethers (estragole, methyl eugenol); Esters; Sesquiterpinols; and Phenols.

Main Body Systems: Immune, respiratory, structural

Physical: Arthritis, cellular terrain balance, chest and lung congestion, chronic fatigue, cold and flu, declutters gut-brain communication, Epstein Barr, fibromyalgia, IBS, joint issues, lymphatic congestion, muscles aches and pains, sinus concerns and toe cramps.

Mental: Anxiety, belief in self, confidence, confusion, depression, happy, headache, lethargy, lifts mood, mental clarity, mental overload, positive outlook, refreshes mind to think clearer, stress and worry.

Emotional: Anguish, despair, discouraged, feel like you have to hide your true self, feel suffocated, grief, identity crisis, introverted, need room to breathe, overburdened, self-acceptance, self-defeating behaviors, shy, trauma.

Chakra: 2nd (sacral), 3rd (solar plexus), 4th (heart), 5th (third eye)

History: Used historically to prevent the spread of disease. Madagacarians consider it their "everything" or "cure all" oil. There has been confusion in the name of Ravintsara, Ravensare, Ho Leaf and Camphor, due to a mis-translation from the Malagasian language. In their country, they call *Cinnamomum camphora*, ravintsara. Although there are similarities in the oil benefits, they are unrelated species. This is why reviewing the botanical name and source is important before employing this oil, to ensure you have what you need to accomplish your purpose in using it *(http://roberttisserand.com/2010/02/ravensara-rant/)* *(http://www.cropwatch.org/RavensaraRavintsara%20Confusion%20Update%201.pdf, http://materiaaromatica.com/default.aspx?go=article&articleID=187)*

Personal Experience: I use this essential oil to combat viral issues such as cold sores and chronic fatigue, respiratory and lung distress, muscle stiffness and mental clutter. Emotionally it has helped during times of grief, sorrow, feeling discouraged and suffocated.

Contraindications: Non-irritating.

Rose *(Rosa damascena)*

Scent: Rich, heavy floral scent with sweet, herbaceous undertones

Note: Middle-Base 7-8

Extraction Method: Steam Distillation (otto); Solvent Extraction (absolute)

Part Used: Flowers

Plant Description: It is a thorny, deciduous shrub that can grow to heights of eight feet. It has oblong, pointed, dark-green leaves with round, multi-layers rose petals in varying colors. It requires lots of moisture in sandy, but well-drained soil, in warm, sunny, wind and cold protected climates. It is a member of the Rosaceae family.

Properties: Analgesic, antibacterial, antidepressant, anti-inflammatory, antiseptic, antiviral, aphrodisiac, astringent, cicatrisant, diuretic, febrifuge, hepatic, sedative, tonic and vulnerary.

Chemistry: Monoterpenols (citronellol, geraniol, nerol, linalool); Sesquiterpenols (farnesol); Monoterpenes (stearoptene, myrcene); Alkanes (nonadecane); Esters (geranyl acetate, neryl acetate); Phenol (eugenol, phenylethanol); and Oxides *(http://www.researchgate.net/publication/232957720_Essential_oil_composition_of_Damask_rose_(Rosa_damascena_Mill.)_distilled_under_different_pressures_and_temperatures)*.

Main Body Systems: Circulation, glandular, hepatic

Physical: Circulation, high blood pressure, hormone imbalances, joint pain, liver stress, menopause, muscle stiffness, PMS, regulate heart rhythm, respiratory distress, rosacea, skin irritations (dry, eczema), sore throat, spleen weakness, tickling cough and women's concerns.

Mental: Anxiety, concentration, depression, distracted easily, exhaustion, hormone headache, insomnia, inspires hope, memory, mental fatigue, optimistic, nervous tension, post-partum depression, PTSD, stress and worry.

Emotional: Anger, betrayal, despair, disappointment, emotionally cold, frustration, grief, insecure about self, irritable, jealousy, joy, low self-esteem, love of self and others, opens the heart to receive, rejection, resentment, sorrow, strengthens spirituality and traumatic emotional wounds.

Chakra: 2nd (sacral), 4th (heart), 6th (third eye), 7th (crown)

History: It has long been revered as a symbol of love and beauty. A Persian scientist, Avicenna, is credited with the invention of the process for extracting rose water from rose petals in the early 11th century. It is said that it takes 60,000 petals to yield just 1 ounce of the oil. Greeks referred to it as "the Queen of Flowers." Romans used in wedding ceremonies and placed rose petals on the marriage bed. It was once a custom to suspend a rose over a dinner or meeting table as a symbol that all confidences uttered around that table would be kept confidential *(http://www.ncbi.nlm.nih.gov/pmc/articles/PMC3586833/)*.

Personal Experience: I use this essential oil in my perfumes, PMS relief, skin and facial products and to combat scarring. Emotionally, it has been versatile in helping with grief, sadness, fear, anger and promoting self-love, acceptance and forgiveness.

Contraindications: Non-irritating.

Rosemary *(Rosmarinus officinalis, verbenone)*

Scent: Camphoraceous, herbaceous, green penetrating, fresh and clean

Note: Middle 6

Extraction Method: Steam distillation

Part Used: Leaves and/or flowers

Plant Description: It is a perennial evergreen shrub that can grow to heights of six feet. It has woody-stemmed branches with silver-green needle-like leaves and small purple flowers. It prefers being in full sun in hydrated but well-drained, calcium-rich soil. It can tolerate maritime weather, but does not transplant well. It is a member of the Labiatae family.

Properties: Analgesic, antibacterial, antifungal, anti-rheumatic, antiseptic, antispasmodic, astringent, cardiotonic, carminative, cephalic, decongestant, diuretic, emmenagogue, hypertensive, insecticide, stimulant and vermifuge.

Chemistry: There are a few chemotypes of rosemary (i.e. ct. 1,8 cineole), so chemistry for each type will vary.

> *ct.1,8 cineole*: Oxides (1,8 cineole); Monoterpenes (pinene, camphene, limonene, myrcene); Ketones (camphone, thujone, verbenone);

Monoterpenols (borneol, terpineol, linalool, terpin-4-ol); Sesquiterpenes (caryophyllene); Esters; and Carboxylic Acids.

Verbenone: Ketones (verbenone, camphor); Monoterpenes (pinene, camphene, limonene); Oxides (1,8 cineole); Esters (bornyl acetate); Monoterpenols (borneol); Carboxylic Acids; and Sesquiterpenes.

Main Body Systems: Circulatory, urinary, structural

Physical: Acne, adrenal support, arthritis, bronchitis, cellulite, cold extremities, dry coughs, gout, hair loss, high cholesterol, increases poor circulation, kidney support, low blood pressure, lymphatic congestion, muscle aches and pains, sinus congestion, skin stagnation, urinary concerns and vein health.

Mental: Alertness, articulate communication, concentration, confidence, creativity, depression, dizziness, exhaustion, focus, forgetfulness, improves memory recall, mental fog and fatigue, negative thoughts, overthinking, rational thinking, self-expression and worry.

Emotional: Betrayal, desire to break free, disconnected from self and spirituality, emotionally stuck, encourages faithfulness and love, feel lost, grounding, infuses joy, opens up heart, overwhelmed, rejection, sadness and trauma from loss.

Chakra: 3rd (solar plexus), 4th (heart), 5th (throat), 6th (third eye)

History: Symbol of love, death and remembrance. Commonly used during the Middle Ages at wedding ceremonies as a "love charm" and at funerals as a sign of remembrance. It was burned in French hospitals to purify the air and prevent infection. Greeks and Romans used it for a variety of medicinal purposes. Commonly used in facial and hair products to stimulate circulation, combat alopecia and open pores.

Personal Experience: I have used this essential oil to stimulate memory and enhance learning, combat sleepiness, muscle fatigue and to soak my tired feet after standing all day. Emotionally it has been good to clear my head, combat emotional congestion and inspire joy, creative and happiness.

Contraindications: Use caution with high blood pressure, epilepsy, heart conditions and during pregnancy.

Rosewood *(Aniba rosaeodora)*

Scent: Woody, herbaceous with hints of sweet, green and floral undertones

Note: Middle to base 7-8

Extraction Method: Steam distillation

Part used: Wood, branches, twigs

Plant Description: It is an evergreen tree that can grow 120 feet tall. It has vibrant green leaves with pointy tips and small clusters of yellow flowers. The bark is reddish and semi-scaly. It prefers moist, but well-drained, acid soil in warm, humid climates. It is a member of the Lauraceae family.

Properties: Analgesic, antibacterial, antidepressant, antifungal, antiseptic, antiviral, aphrodisiac, cephalic, cytophylactic, deodorant, insecticide, sedating while stimulating and tonic.

Chemistry: Monoterpenols (linalool, terpineol, geraniol); Oxides (1,8 cineole, linalool oxide); Monoterpenes (pinene, camphene, myrcene, limonene); Sesquiterpenes (copaene); Aldehydes (neral, geranial, benzaldehyde); and Ketones.

Main Body Systems: Immune, nervous, structural

Physical: Acne, bronchitis, chronic fatigue, dry cough, fibromyalgia, hormone balancing, laryngitis, muscle fatigue, neuralgia, skin tonic (mature, wrinkles, dry, sensitive, damaged), spleen support and urinary concerns.

Mental: Anxiety, calms the mind, contentment, depression, exhaustion, headaches, insomnia, jet lag, meditation, mental fatigue, nervous tension, open-mindedness, over-analytical, overwhelmed by circumstances, stress and weary.

Emotional: Abandonment, calms heated emotions, comforts the heart, emotional balance, feel exploited and taken advantage of, frigidity, grief, inner peace, inner strength, judgmental, overburdened, overwhelmed, rejection, self-love, spiritual freedom and tolerant of challenges.

Chakra: 1st (root), 2nd (sacral), 4th (heart)

History: Amazonians used the wood to make canoes, furniture, cabinetry and other wood structures. It has been used extensively in perfumeries. Due to over-exploitation and poor harvesting practices, it has become an endangered tree. To combat its extinction, the Brazilian government enacted legislation requiring distilleries to plant a new tree for each one it cuts down.

Personal Experience: I use this essential oil in my skin care to nourish and hydrate skin, to combat urinary issues and promote mental awareness. Emotionally it instills an inner peace, contentment and acceptance without feeling overburdened.

Contraindications: Non-irritating.

Sage *(Salvia officinalis)*

Scent: Fresh, herbaceous and sweet with camphor undertones

Note: Middle 7

Extraction Method: Steam distillation

Part used: Leaves

Plant Description: It is an herbaceous, evergreen shrub that can grow up to two feet tall. It has silvery-green, fuzzy, cone-shaped leaves with clusters of small purple flowers. It prefers warm climates, in the sun (does not do well in the shade) with well-drained but hydrated soil. It is drought and frost tolerant. It is a member of the Labiatae family.

Properties: Antibacterial, antifungal, antigalactagogue, anti-inflammatory, antioxidant, antiseptic, antispasmodic, astringent, carminative, cholagogue, choleretic, cicatrisant, deodorant, depurative, digestive, emmenagogue, febrifuge, stimulant, tonic and vasodilator.

Chemistry: Ketones (thujone, camphor); Monoterpenes (camphene, pinene, myrcene, limonene, cymene); Monoterpenols (linalool, borneol, terpineol, terpin-4-ol); Sesquiterpenols (viridiflorol); Oxides (1,8 cineole); Sesquiterpenes (humulene, caryophyllene); Esters (bornyl acetate, linalyl acetate); Ethers (estragole); and Diterpenols.

Main Body Systems: Lymphatic, respiratory, urinary

Physical: Arthritis and joint pain, colds, dental health, edema, excessive sweating, salivation and urination, nail fungus, indigestion, intestinal parasites, kidney and liver purifier, lymphatic sluggishness, muscle and nerve tremors, night sweats, PMS, respiratory distress, sore throat and yeast issues.

Mental: Anxiety, cleanses mental clutter, dispels negativity, fatigue, forgetful, headaches, hyperactive, inflexible thinking, mental clarity, mental harmony, nervousness and rapid thoughts.

Emotional: Aura purification, enhance inner knowing, feel held back by clutter, grief, guilt, hysteria, lack of emotional stability, self-acceptance of true identity, shock, trauma and vulnerability.

Chakra: 1st (root), 4th (heart), 5th (throat), 6th (third eye)

History: Ancient physicians used sage as a diuretic, hemostatic and emmenagogue. Greeks used for liver issues and as a memory enhancer. Egyptians used to combat the plague and gave to women who had a difficult time getting pregnant. It is also a popular choice in culinary dishes for its taste and preservative qualities.

Personal Experience: I use this essential oil for lymphatic and urinary stagnation, to purify the air and mental congestion. It helps me combat negative energy and thoughts as well as purify my spirit to allow the fun side to come out.

Contraindications: Avoid during pregnancy, breastfeeding, epilepsy and seizures.

Sandalwood *(Santalum album, spicatum)*

Scent: Woodsy, honey-like with sweet, earthy and exotic undertones

Note: Base 8-9

Extraction Method: Steam distillation

Part used: Wood

Plant Description: It is a parasitic tree, surviving off its surrounding trees that can grow up to 45 feet tall. It has a slender trunk with silver-brown, flexible branches with dark-green, oval, glossy leaves and green and purple berries. The heartwood can take up to 20 years before distillation of the essential oil, and up to 80 years before full maturity. It prefers warm, sunny areas in alkaline soil. It does not grow well in the shade or moist climates. It is a member of the Santalaceae family.

Properties: Antibacterial, antidepressant, anti-inflammatory, antiparasitic, antiseptic, antispasmodic, antiviral, aphrodisiac, astringent, carminative, diuretic, expectorant, sedative and tonic.

Chemistry: Sesquiterpenols (santalol, farnesol); Sesquiterpenes (santalene); Esters (santyl acetate); and Carboxylic Acids (santalic acid).

Main Body Systems: Respiratory, structural, urinary

Physical: Acne, arthritis and joint pain, dry coughs, laryngitis, lung concerns, lymphatic congestion, PMS, respiratory ailments, skin irritations (eczema mature, rashes), urinary issues and tooth and gum health.

Mental: Ability to adapt to varying situations, anxiety, codependence, confusion, creativity, depression, indecisive, headaches, helps people put all of the pieces together to see the bigger picture, insomnia, keeps feet on the ground to stay focused, meditation, nervous tension, relaxation, stress and worry.

Emotional: Anger, compares self to others, feel isolated, grief, grounding, inflexibility, inner connectedness, insecurity, rage, rejection, searching for true identity, self-acceptance, strength with parasitic relationship, stuck in the past and worthlessness.

Chakra: 1st (root), 2nd (sacral), 3rd (solar plexus), 4th (heart), 5th (throat)

History: Ayurveda medicine used it for kidney, bladder and respiratory ailments. Tibetan medicine used for emotional weariness during times of excessive mental exertion. It has long been used as a fixative in perfumes and incenses. Egyptians employed in the embalming process. Widely used in religious ceremonies in India. Chinese medicine uses it to improve digestive heat and relieve pain. Due to over-exploitation, it is becoming more endangered.

Personal Experience: I use this essential oil for sore throats, dry coughs, laryngitis, lymphatic and urinary congestion. Emotionally, it helps me see the bigger picture, opening my eyes and mind to all possibilities with courage and inner strength.

Contraindications: Non-irritating.

Savory *(Satureia montana, Satureia hortense)*

Scent: Earthy, herbaceous, green with slight bitter and camphoraceous undertones

Note: Middle 6

Extraction Method: Steam Distillation

Part Used: Leaves

Plant Description: It is a short, compact and hardy, semi-evergreen perennial plant that spreads out when it grows to heights of one to two feet. It has woody stems at its base with small, oblong, dark-green leaves and small, light purple flowers. It prefers hydrated but well-drained chalky soil in sunny areas. It is a member of the Labiatae family.

Properties: Antibacterial, antifungal, anti-inflammatory, antiparasitic, antiseptic, antiviral, aphrodisiac, astringent, carminative, decongestant, diaphoretic, expectorant, stimulant, stomachic and vermifuge.

Chemistry: Phenol (carvacrol, thymol, carvacrol methyl ether); Monoterpenes (cymene, terpinene, pinene); Monoterpenols (linalool, terpineol); Sesquiterpenes (caryophyllene); Oxides (1,8 cineole); and Ketones.

Main Body Systems: Digestion, immune, intestinal

Physical: Bronchitis, candida, colds and flu, fever, earaches, Helicobacter pylori, IBS, indigestion, intestinal issues, nasal congestion with drainage, respiratory ailments, rheumatism, sciatica and sore throat.

Mental: Anxiety, confidence, control, deep thought, exhaustion, inflexible thoughts, lethargy, listen to inner senses and voice when decision making, mental fatigue, mood swings, nervousness, sharpen the mind and worry.

Emotional: Agoraphobia, defensive when personal space is invaded, fear of intimacy, feel inadequate, need to feel protected, savoring ones gifts, sensitive to criticism, stability, security, warms cold emotions and withdrawn emotionally.

Chakra: 2nd (sacral), 3rd (solar plexus), 4th (heart)

History: Greeks used it as an aphrodisiac. Romans used in culinary dishes to stimulate digestion. Early physicians used for colic, poor elimination and rheumatism. Used in love potions to savor love and relationships. Ancient and modern times use for bee and wasp sting discomfort.

Personal Experience: I use this essential oil to enhance digestion, calm intestinal upset and for earaches. Emotionally it has helped during times I feel defensive, unappreciated and unworthy.

Contraindications: Can be irritating in large amounts.

Spearmint *(Mentha spicata, cardiaca)*

Scent: Minty, refreshing, uplifting, camphoraceous with sweet undertones

Note: Middle 6

Extraction Method: Steam Distillation

Part Used: Leaves and/or flowers

Plant Description: It is a perennial plant that can grow to heights of three feet tall. It has ribbed, vibrant green, small leaves and produces pale purple flowers. It prefers warm climates with semi-shade in dry, sandy, acid and hydrated soil. It is a member of the Labiatae family.

Properties: Analgesic, antibacterial, antifungal, antigalactagogue, anti-inflammatory, antiseptic, antispasmodic, antiviral, astringent, carminative, decongestant, expectorant, febrifuge, hepatic, nervine, stimulant, sudorific and tonic.

Chemistry: Ketones (carvone, dihydrocarvone, menthone); Monoterpenes (limonene, myrcene, camphene); Monoterpenols (carveol, linalool, thujanol, octanol); Sesquiterpenes (caryophyllene); Esters (carvyl acetate); Oxides (1,8 cineole); Sesquiterpinols; and Phenols.

Main Body Systems: Digestive, respiratory, structural

Physical: Acne (blackheads), allergies, bronchitis, body aches during cold and flu, GI upset, headaches, hot flashes, IBS, indigestion, kidney fatigue, nausea, night sweats, painful urination, PMS, sciatica, sinus congestion and toothaches.

Mental: Adapt to change and new environments, anxiety, alertness, concentration, confidence, depression, exhaustion, fatigue, focus, grief, guilt, headaches, lethargy, lifts spirits, mental clarity, nervous tension, perfectionist, reduces stress and refreshes a tired mind.

Emotional: Anger, believe in self, bitterness, cheerful, combat extreme shyness, defensive, frustration, inner strength, inspires a playful personality, irritability, jealousy, joy, quarrelsome, rage, repression to avoid conflict, resentment, self-esteem, stand up for self and trauma.

Chakra: 2nd (sacral), 3rd (solar plexus), 5th (throat), 6th (third eye)

History: Used often in culinary dishes for flavor and as a digestive aid. Ancient Greeks used to restore the mind and body as well in bath water for rejuvenation. Medieval times used for oral hygiene, sore gums and as a teeth whitener.

Personal Experience: I use this essential oil for headaches, digestive upset, nerve pain and respiratory distress. Emotionally, it helps open my mind with clarity and focus, look at a situation with "fresh eyes" and feel freedom to dream without constraints.

Contraindications: Dilute in a carrier as it may cause skin irritation. Avoid during breastfeeding.

Spikenard (*Nardostachys chinensis, grandiflora, jatamansi*)

Scent: Earthy and herbaceous with hints of sweet and pungent undertones

Note: Base 9-10

Extraction Method: Steam Distillation

Part Used: Root

Plant Description: It is a perennial plant that grows one to three feet tall. It has dark green, heart-shaped leaves with serrated edges and small white-pink flowers. It has a woody stem system and root system. It prefers sandy, alkaline and moist soil and semi-shade to no shade. It is a member of the Valerianaceae family.

Properties: Antibacterial, anti-inflammatory, antispasmodic, antiviral, cardiotonic, carminative, deodorant, diuretic, emmenagogue, nervine, sedative and stomachic.

Chemistry: Sesquiterpenes (gurjunene, maalene, aristoladiene, aristolene, seychellene); Monoterpenes (carlarene, ionene, pinene); Sesquiterpenols (patchoulol, nardol); Ketones (aristolenone, ionone); Aldehydes (valerianal); Coumarins; Oxides (1,8 cineole); Esters (bornyl acetate); and Carboxylic Acids.

Main Body Systems: Glandular, nervous, respiratory

Physical: Back pain, bronchitis, dry, hacking cough, heart health, hemorrhoids, indigestion, kidney and liver deficiencies, PMS, muscle spasms, nerve pain, nervous stomach, skin irritations and vein health.

Mental: Anxiety, calms mental overload, confidence, confusion, indecisive, depression, focus, grounding, headache, insomnia, inspiration, nervous tension, panic, restless, stress and worry.

Emotional: Anger, comforting, connect to self, deep emotional wounds, despair, emotional balance, encourages humility, heartache, hopelessness, hysteria, inner knowing, inner strength, keeps feet on the ground, overwhelmed by emotion, peace, shock, trauma and weepiness.

Chakra: 1st (root), 2nd (sacral), 4th (heart), 5th (throat), 7th (crown)

History: A fixative in ancient Greek and Roman perfumes, as well as still used today. Egyptians and Indians used for both spiritual and medicinal purposes. Native Americans used the root in a tea for backaches. The bible tells of Mary Magdalene anointing Jesus' feet with spikenard prior to the Last Supper.

Personal Experience: I use this essential oil to keep my feet and mind on the ground. Emotionally it has calmed my nerves, made me feel stable and capable of managing stressful situations. It is great for spiritual connection and mediation.

Contraindications: Non-irritating.

Spruce *(Tsuga Canadensis, Picea sitka, alba)* Black Spruce *(Picea mariana)*

Scent: Woody, herbaceous, fresh with camphoraceous undertones

Note: Middle 7

Extraction Method: Steam Distillation

Part Used: Needles

Plant Description: There are several species of Spruce grown all over the world. It is a pyramidal evergreen tree that typically grows between 30-65 feet tall. It has layered branches with short, silver-green needs leaves and brown, oval cones. It prefers moist but well-drained, sandy, acid soil in full sun to semi-shade. They burn quickly in fires, but spread seeds post-fire to repopulate. It is a member of the Pinaceae family.

Properties: Analgesic, antibacterial, antifungal, antiseptic, antiviral, astringent, decongestant, diaphoretic, diuretic, expectorant, nervine, respiratory tonic, rubefacient, stimulant and styptic.

Chemistry: Hemlock is more monoterpene rich whereas Black Spruce is more ester rich.

Monoterpenes (camphene, pinene, limonene, phellandrene, myrcene); Esters (Bornyl acetate); Sesquiterpenes (tricyclene, dipentene, cadinene); Ketones (carvone, thujone); and Monoterpinol (borneol).

Main Body Systems: Digestion, respiratory, urinary

Physical: Acne, adrenal support, arthritis, asthma, blood sugar balance, bronchitis, cold and flu, colitis, deep breathing, diarrhea, GI ailments, gingivitis, hemorrhoids, kidney strengthener, respiratory congestion, skin irritations (eczema, rash), sore throats and vein health.

Mental: Anxiety, cognitive strength, concentration, confusion, creative freedom, fatigue, focus, hopeful, optimistic, mental clarity, mood swings, nervous, panic, self-doubt, stress, uplifting and worry.

Emotional: Ability to stand up for self with compassion, betrayal, despair, embrace the bigger picture of a challenging situation, feel nurtured, grief, grounding, resilience to recover after being "burned" by a friend, self-acceptance, sorrow and suffocating emotions.

Chakra: 1st (root), 4th (heart), 5th (throat), 7th (crown)

History: Historically shown to possess vitamin C thus used in ancient cultures for respiratory and immune issues. Native North American Indian tribes used it for lung issues and wounds due to its antiseptic properties, as well as the strong, flexible limbs for making baskets.

Personal Experience: I use this essential oil for respiratory congestion and to enhance deep breathing especially with bronchitis, for urinary and digestive weakness. Emotionally it gives me space to think and feel without being burdened or feeling guilty.

Contraindications: Non-irritating.

St John's Wort *(Hypericum perforatum)*

Scent: Earthy, woody, pungent with slight sweet undertones

Note: Middle 6-7

Extraction Method: Steam Distillation

Part Used: Leaves and flowers

Plant Description: It is a hardy, perennial plant that can grow up to three feet tall. It has narrow, oblong, medium green leaves along the stem, yellow, star-like flowers with many stamens at the center and creeping rhizomes. It prefers sandy, acid, moist but well-drained soil in sun and partial shade. It is a member of the Hypericaceae family.

Properties: Analgesic, antidepressant, anti-inflammatory, antiparasitic, antiseptic, antispasmodic, antiviral, astringent, cholagogue, diuretic, hepatic, nervine, sedative and vulnerary.

Chemistry: Monoterpenes (pinene, myrcene, limonene); Sesquiterpenes (caryophyllene, humulene, germacrene); Monoterpenols (terpineol, geraniol,); Oxides (caryophyllene oxide); Alkanes (decane, nonane); and Phenols (*http://www.ncbi.nlm.nih.gov/pmc/articles/PMC2975376/, http://jocpr.com/vol2-iss6-2010/JCPR-2010-2-6-284-290.pdf*).

Main Body Systems: Intestinal, glandular, nervous

Physical: Bladder issues, bronchitis, bruises, colds and viruses, diarrhea, female imbalances, fibromyalgia, gall bladder, liver and lung support, IBS, neuropathy, rheumatism, sciatica, skin irritations (burns, eczema, dry skin), toothaches, ulcers and wounds.

Mental: Addictions, anxiety, dark thoughts, depression, insomnia, negative thinking, mental chatter, mood stabilizer, nervousness, panic attacks, racing thoughts, Seasonal Affective Disorder (SAD), stress, tension headaches and worry.

Emotional: Anger, betrayal, bitterness, deep emotional wounds, emotional confusion, fear, feel attacked and overwhelmed by circumstances, heart-broken, hysteria, PTSD, resentment, self-worth, shock, stabbed in the back, trauma and victimized.

Chakra: 1st (root), 3rd (solar plexus), 4th (heart), 6th (third eye)

History: Very common among Greeks for nervous disorders. Hippocrates used it for intestinal worms. Folklore connects St. John's Wort with John the Baptist, whose birthday is June 24, coinciding with the time St. John's Wort blooms. Today, it is most noted for its benefits with depression, mood and PTSD.

Personal Experience: I use this essential oil for mental and emotional stability as it worked wonderfully for anxiety, depression and PTSD. It can quiet an overactive mind with racing thoughts. It has also been a staple in my intestinal and nervous system blends, also combating my nerve pain and skin irritations.

Contraindications: With some prescription medications such as antidepressants and birth control, so cross-reference the precautions. Avoid during pregnancy due to its abortive properties. Photosensitive.

Tanacetum annuum (Blue Tansy)

Scent: Rich, fruity-sweet, herbaceous earthy undertones

Note: Middle to Base 7-8

Extraction Method: Steam Distillation

Part Used: Leaves and Flowers

Plant Description: It is an herbaceous plant that can grow up to three feet tall. It has dark green, feathery leaves with clusters of hardy, round, medium yellow colored flowers. It prefers sandy, well-drained soil in the sun, as it does not fare well in the shade. It is wind and frost tolerant, but maritime tender. It is a member of the Compositae family.

Properties: Antibacterial, antifungal, anti-histamine, anti-inflammatory, antispasmodic, antiviral, carminative, febrifuge, insecticide, sedative and stimulant simultaneously, tonic, vermifuge and vulnerary.

Chemistry: Monoterpenes (sabinene, myrcene, limonene, pinene, phellandrene, cymene); Sesquiterpenes (chamazulene, dihydrochamazulene); Ketones (camphor, thujone, artemisone, camphone, isopinocamphone, piperitone); Monoterpenols (borneol); Sesquiterpenols (farnesene); and Oxides.

Main Body Systems: Glandular, nervous, structural

Physical: Adrenal support, excess mucus, endocrine system support, IBS and intestinal upset, lice and fleas, kidney issues, neuralgia, PMS, roseacea, skin irritations (eruptions, eczema, scabies), thyroid support and vein health.

Mental: Accepting, anxiety, depression, confusion, exhaustion, focus, memory recall, mental fatigue, moody, multi-tasking facilitator, nervousness, and self-confidence, tension and worry.

Emotional: Anger, bury feelings to protect others, defensive from attack, frustration, grief, hysteria, invasion of boundaries, irritability, need to be taken care of, shock, smothered and trauma.

Chakra: 1st (crown), 2nd (sacral), 4th (heart), 5th (throat), 7th (crown)

History: Greeks used it for medicinal purposes, 8th Century AD Swiss used for intestinal worms, rheumatism, digestive problems and fevers. 19th Century Irish used for joint pain. During the 19th Century, the English placed tansy among the deceased for its worm warding benefits. In 2008, Sweden researchers investigated the use of tansy to repel ticks, showing a 64–72% repellency.

Personal Experience: This is one of my favorite essential oils for adrenal support and nourishment (along with mandarin, pine and Roman chamomile). It calms my mind, quiets racing thoughts and helps me gain perspective with a positive outlook. It has also helped to combat inflammation, PMS spasms and intestinal upset.

Contraindications: May cause skin irritation if undiluted. May stain clothing and fabrics.

Tangerine *(Citrus reticulata)* – See Orange

Tarragon *(Artemisia dracunculus)*

Scent: Licorice scent with herbaceous undertones

Note: Middle to Base 7-8 (1 drop can be powerful in a blend)

Extraction Method: Steam Distillation

Part Used: Leaves

Plant Description: It is an herbaceous plant that can grow up to three feet tall and spreads with runners. It has long, narrow, dark green leaves with a wooden stem and small, vibrant yellow flowers that do not usually open fully. It prefers sandy, alkaline, moist but well-drained soil in semi-shade to no shade. It is drought tolerant. It is a member of the Compositae family.

Properties: Analgesic, antibacterial, antifungal, antiparasitic, antiseptic, antioxidant, antiviral, deodorant, digestive, diuretic, febrifuge, insecticide, stimulant, stomachic and vermifuge.

Chemistry: Ethers (estragole, trans-anethole, methyl eugenol); Monoterpenes (ocimene, limonene, pinene, camphene, phellandrene); Monoterpenols (nerol); Coumarins (herniarin); Oxides (1,8 cineole); and Ketones (thujone).

Main Body Systems: Digestive, intestinal, urinary

Physical: Arthritis, digestive concerns, dry cough, E.coli, edema, fatigue, heart palpitations, immune weakness, intestinal parasites, neuromuscular spasms, physical debility, PMS, sciatica, weeping wounds (skin irritations), PMS, staph infections and toothaches.

Mental: Addiction, authoritative, defeated, determination, inspires passion and drive, mental fatigue, self-confidence, sluggish thinking, surrender to being overpowered and willpower.

Emotional: Abandonment, abusive past, been treated like a dog, disappointment, emotionally wounded, fear, jealousy, over-nurturer and sacrifice self, self-respect, self-worth, violent tendencies and vulnerable.

Chakra: 1st (root), 3rd (solar plexus), 5th (throat)

History: Its botanical name translates to "little dragon", which can be analyzed as being beneficial in combat – physically, mentally and emotionally. Used by herbalists for head, heart and liver ailments. Pliny, a Roman scholar considered tarragon beneficial for fatigue. Used often in culinary dishes, to flavor vinegar and soups (*http://www.ncbi.nlm.nih.gov/pmc/articles/PMC3391558/*).

Personal Experience: I love this essential oil for emotional and mental strength (especially during "battles"), and to help me when I feel defeated and overpowered. Physically it has helped with intestinal parasites, digestive upset, nerve pain, general fatigue and overall weakness.

Contraindications: Use sparingly when using with children and during pregnancy due to its methyl chavicol content.

Tea Tree *(Melaleuca alternifolia)*

Scent: Camphoraceous, pungent, fresh, clean scent with spicy undertones

Note: Middle 6-7

Extraction Method: Steam Distillation

Part Used: Leaves

Plant Description: It is an evergreen shrub that can grow up to twenty feet tall. It has long, narrow, dark green, sprig-like leaves with fuzzy-like flowers in which the plethora of stamens form the shape of a round brush. It prefers sandy, acid and moist but well-drained soil in full sun, as it does not like the shade. It is a member of the Myrtaceae family.

Properties: Analgesic, antibacterial, antibiotic, antifungal, antiparasitic, antiseptic, antiviral, cicatrisant, decongestant, deodorant, diaphoretic, disinfectant, expectorant, immune stimulant, insecticide and vermifuge.

Chemistry: Monoterpenes (terpinene, pinene, cymene, sabinene, myrcene, phellandrene, limonene); Phenols (terpin-4-ol); Monoterpenols (terpineol); Sesquiterpenes (cadinene, aromadrene, viridiflorene); Oxides (1,8 cineole, 1,4 cineole); and Sesquiterpenols (globulol).

Main Body Systems: Intestinal, respiratory, structural

Physical: Bronchitis, cold and flu, cold sores, cough, dandruff, fever blisters, fungal issues (nail, skin, candida), herpes simplex, insect bites, lice and fleas, mold, muscle aches and pains, respiratory ailments and skin irritations (acne, rashes, ringworm, scrapes, wounds).

Mental: Creativity, dispels negativity, lethargy, lifts spirit, mentally overwhelmed, refreshes the mind, promotes a positive outlook, self-confidence booster, stress reduction and worrying too much.

Emotional: Attacked, emotional wounds, feel consumed by responsibilities, sharp emotions, smothered, shock, struggle, suffocated, tough to recover after hardships, trauma and victimized.

Chakra: 1st (root), 3rd (solar plexus), 5th (throat), 6th (third eye)

History: During World War I, Australian soldiers used tea tree to disinfectant their wounds. Numerous research studies have been conducted on tea tree, especially since the 1920's when the Australian government discovered its potent and effective therapeutic properties. It is most popular for its antimicrobial and antifungal properties, dispelling environmental mold and fungus, yeast and candida (http://www.ncbi.nlm.nih.gov/pubmed/26042369).

Personal Experience: I love this essential oil for most skin issues, fungal concerns (like nail fungus, especially when combined with patchouli) and to enhance the respiratory system. Emotionally, I have found it to inspire and open my mind, provoke positivity and help me breathe through a situation when I feel attacked or like things are caving in.

Contraindications: Can be sensitizing to the skin for some people after long-term use. Use caution with internal applications. Common allergies to melaleuca.

161

Thyme *(Thymus vulgaris)*

Scent: Fresh, herbaceous, green, penetrating scent

Note: Middle 7

Extraction Method: Steam Distillation

Part Used: Leaves and/or flowers

Plant Description: It is an evergreen shrub that can grow up to one foot tall. It has small, clusters of dark-green leaves and small, purple flowers. It prefers well-drained, alkaline, clay or limestone-like soil in the sun, as it does not like the shade. It is frost and mild wind tolerant. It is a member of the Labiatae family.

Properties: Antibacterial, antifungal, antiparasitic, antiseptic, antispasmodic, antiviral, astringent, carminative, disinfectant, diuretic, expectorant, febrifuge, insecticide, nervine, purgative, stimulant and tonic.

Chemistry: There are numerous chemotypes for thyme (i.e., ct. thymol, ct. linalool and ct. carvacrol), so chemistry will vary per type. Monoterpenols (linalool, terpin-4-ol, thujanol, geraniol); Monoterpenes (myrcene, cymene, terpinene, thujene); Sesquiterpenes (caryophyllene); Phenols (thymol, carvacrol); and Esters (linalyl acetate).

Main Body Systems: Digestive, intestinal, respiratory

Physical: Alopecia, asthma, bronchitis, circulation, cold and flu, cough (dry and whooping), diarrhea, gastritis, gout, gum health, immune strength, intestinal parasites, laryngitis, low blood pressure, lung and respiratory support, muscle aches, PMS cramps, sore throat and sluggish metabolism.

Mental: Alert, concentration, depression, introversion, invigorate purpose, mental clarity, mental exhaustion, motivation, nervous, refreshing, stress, vasodilative headaches and vigor.

Emotional: Courage, endure challenges, emotionally cold, emotional stamina, frustration, grief, guilt, impulsive reactions, overshadowed, room to breathe, suffocated, suppressed and trouble digesting a circumstance.

Chakra: 1st (root), 3rd (solar plexus), 5th (throat), 6th (third eye)

History: Medicinally it dates as far back as 3500 BC and has long been used as a digestive aid (indigestion and flatulence) and a remedy for epilepsy. In ancient and medieval times, this plant was thought to inspire bravery. Thyme, clove and lemon were used as a disinfectant in hospitals prior WWI. Commonly added to food dishes for taste and digestive support.

Personal Experience: I love this essential oil for any digestive or intestinal support, respiratory concerns and circulation stimulator (especially with cold hands and feet). Emotionally it refreshes my mind while connecting me to the earth, motivates me and helps me not feel overwhelmed by situations.

Contraindications: Use caution with high blood pressure and excess heated health concerns.

Turmeric *(Curcuma longa)*

Scent: Rich, spicy, earthy, herbaceous with peppery and semi-sweet undertones

Note: Middle 7

Extraction Method: Carbon Dioxide, Steam Distillation

Part Used: Rhizomes (roots)

Plant Description: It is a rhizomatous, perennial herb that can grow up to three feet tall. It has hardy, bright green, long, smooth, floppy leaves with a pineapple-shaped cluster of white-pink flowers. It has hardy rhizomes of which the essential oil is produced. It prefers acidic, moist but well-drained soil in wet climates with sun or partial shade. It is a member of the Zingiberaceae family.

Properties: Analgesic, antibacterial, antidiarrheal, anti-inflammatory, anti-parasitic, antioxidant, antiviral, astringent, cardiotonic, carminative, cholagogue, depurative, febrifuge, hepatic, insecticide, nutritive, stomachic and vulnerary.

Chemistry: Ketone (turmerone, atlantone); Sesquiterpene (bisabolene, zingiberene) Oxides (1,8 cineole); Monoterpenols (borneol); Monoterpenes (cymene, pinene, myrcene, phellandrene); Sesquiterpenes (terpinolene); Phenols (curcuphenol); and Ketones (carvacrol) *(http://220.227.138.214:8080/dspace/bitstream/123456789/255/1/Chemical+Composition.PDF)*.

Main Body Systems: Circulatory, hepatic, structural

Physical: Allergies, bronchitis, cardiovascular issues (blood pressure, cholesterol, triglycerides), diabetes, digestive and intestinal concerns, edema, heartburn, hemorrhoids, IBS, liver support, muscle aches and pains, osteoarthritis, skin issues (itching, irritation, eczema), TMJ and wounds.

Mental: Anxiety, concentration, creative, depression, fatigue, focus, jittery, memory recall, mental stamina, performance, PTSD, restless, self-confidence, sluggish, stress, willpower and worry.

Emotional: Anger, attacked and defenseless, bitterness, despair, disappointment, emotional congestion, fear, feel oversaturated, frustration, impatient, inflexible, irritability, sensitive to criticism and worthiness.

Chakra: 2nd (sacral), 3rd (solar plexus), 4th (heart)

History: It is a popular spice, especially in Indian cuisine, as an ingredient of curry powder. It has a deep orange-yellow color and contains high amounts of curcumin, scientifically shown to possess powerful anti-inflammatory properties. In India, turmeric has been used as a remedy for stomach and liver ailments. The robes of the Hindu monks were traditionally colored with a yellow dye made of turmeric, as well as Indonesians dyed their bodies as part of their wedding ritual. In Thailand, turmeric rhizomes have been used for dizziness and peptic ulcers.

Personal Experience: I love this oil to combat inflammation anywhere in the body, digestive support, skin issues, sore muscles and joint pain. It provides an emotional strength to handle heated situations and endure tough times.

Contraindications: Mild to non-irritating.

Vanilla *(Vanilla planifolia)*

Scent: Sweet, rich, balsamic, bourbon-like with herbaceous and spicy undertones

Note: Middle to Base 7-8

Extraction Method: Carbon Dioxide

Part Used: Bean

Plant Description: It is an orchid and a thick, evergreen vine that climbs and attaches to tree trunks and other supports by its fleshy roots, growing up to 100 feet tall. It has thick, oblong, dark green leaves and green-yellow trumpet-shaped flowers, which last only one day and must be hand-pollinated (in the morning) to produce a seedpod, the "vanilla bean". The pods grow to be about 6-9 inches long. It prefers moist soil in hot, wet and tropical climates. It is a member of the Orchidaceae family.

Properties: Antibacterial, antidepressant, anti-inflammatory, antioxidant, antispasmodic, aphrodisiac, carminative, emmenagogue, febrifuge, sedative and vulnerary.

Chemistry: Aldehydes (vanillin, hydroxybenzaldehyde, piperonal); Carboxylic Acids (vanillic acid, hydroxybenzoic acid, hexanoic acid); and Phenol (eugenol).

Main Body Systems: Digestion, glandular, nervous

Physical: Carbohydrate metabolism, digestive aid, high blood pressure, hormone balance, immune system support, libido, muscle spasms, nausea, performance, PMS and vein health.

Mental: Alertness, anxiety, calms nerves, concentration, indecisive, depression, insomnia, mental clarity and stamina, nervous, panic attacks, stress and worry.

Emotional: Anger, co-dependent, comforting, emotional fatigue, feel attacked, forgiveness, grief, loneliness, needy, security, self-love, trauma and warms cold emotions.

Chakra: 1st (root), 2nd (sacral), 3rd (solar plexus), 4th (heart), 6th (third eye)

History: Native legends say that vanilla was introduced to Cortez by Montezuma in 1520 and then to Europe by Cortez. It was used by the Aztecs to flavor their royal drink xocolatl (a mixture of cocoa beans, vanilla and honey). Ancient Africa used for stomach ailments and 16th century Europe used for stomach poisoning. It is a popular ingredient in food dishes, desserts and beverages. And a popular scent in the perfume industry, Francois Coty made famous in his 1927 perfume, L'Aimant. Used in some manufacturing of pharmaceuticals (i.e. L-dopa for Parkinson's), *(http://articles.mercola.com/herbal-oils/vanilla-oil.aspx)*.

Personal Experience: I love this essential oil to warm my emotions, bring comfort, joy and relaxation to my mind. Physically, it has been helpful for vein and digestive health.

Contraindications: Non-irritating.

Vetiver (*Vetivera zizanioides, Andropogen muricatus*)

Scent: Deep, earthy, heavy, smoky yet clean with semi-sweet, spicy undertones

Note: Base 9-10

Extraction Method: Steam Distillation

Part Used: Root

Plant Description: It is a tall, erect but weepy grass (similar to lemongrass) that can grow up to five feet tall. The light green leaves are long and, narrow, stern at the base and weepy at the ends, flopping over. The roots are clustered in long, skinny strands. It prefers dry, clay, alkaline soil in warm, sunny climates, as it is frost sensitive. It is a member of the Poaceae family.

Properties: Antibacterial, anti-inflammatory, antioxidant, antispasmodic, antiviral, antiseptic, cytophylactic, hepatic, nervine, sedative, tonic, vermifuge and vulnerary.

Chemistry: Sesquiterpenols (isovalencinol, bicyclovetinerol, khusenol, vetiverol); Ketones (vitivone, khusimone, nootkatone); Sesquiterpenes; Esters (vetiveryl acetate); and Carboxylic Acids (benzoic acid, vetivenic acid).

Main Body Systems: Glandular, nervous, structural

Physical: Alopecia, blood purifier, cools liver issues, coughs (dry), indigestion, intestinal spasms, hormone balance, hot flashes, laryngitis, muscle aches, physical performance, PMS and skin concerns (mature, dry, wrinkles, stretch marks, rosacea).

Mental: Anxiety, articulation, concentration, confusion, dementia, focus, exhaustion, fatigue, headaches, hysteria, insomnia, lack of purpose and direction, learning ability, mental strength, nervous, neurotic behavior, overactive mind, oversensitivity, perfectionist, promote positivity, stress and tension.

Emotional: Anger, betrayal, emotional burnout, emotional harmony, feeling unworthy, fragile, frustration, jealousy, self-grounding, speaking up for self with confidence, spiritual calmness, strengthen self-identity and vulnerable.

Chakra: 1st (root), 2nd (sacral), 3rd (solar plexus), 5th (throat), 7th (crown)

History: Its roots are considered to be an emblem of vitality. It has long been a fixative in many perfumes and colognes. In Asia, the roots are woven into coarse mats and hung in front of the doors. The roots from which the thick, amber essential oil is distilled have long been used to prevent soil erosion (and potential heavy metal contamination in groundwater *(http://www.ncbi.nlm.nih.gov/pubmed/24409635)*, *http://www.sciencedirect.com/science/article/pii/S0883292704000587)*.

Personal Experience: I love this essential oil for skin and respiratory issues. It is very grounding, calms mental chatter and confusion and promotes a feeling of strength during challenges with an "I can handle this" attitude.

Contraindications: Non-irritating.

Violet (*Viola odorata*)

Scent: Sweet, floral, green, clean with herbaceous undertones

Note: Middle 7

Extraction Method: Solvent Expression

Part Used: Leaves and/or flowers

Plant Description: It is a perennial evergreen shrub that is low-lying to the ground, reaching heights up to six inches high. It has dark green, heart-shaped leaves with small deep blue-ish purple flowers. It prefers cool, moist but well-drained, sandy soil in sunny but shades areas, as it doesn't like the hot winds or frost. It is a member of the Violaceae family.

Properties: Analgesic, antibacterial, anti-inflammatory, antioxidant, antispasmodic, antiviral, antiseptic, aphrodisiac, cardiotonic, demulcent, diaphoretic, febrifuge, hepatic, relaxant and vulnerary.

Chemistry: Monoterpenols (linalool, terpin-4-ol); Sesquiterpenols (cadinol, globulol, viridiflorol, cubenol, ledol); Ketone (1-Phenyl butanone, pugelone); Sesquiterpenes (germacrene, Viridiflorene); and Esters (benzyl benzoate) *(http://scholarsresearchlibrary.com/aasr-vol3-iss5/AASR-2011-3-5-44-51.pdf)*.

Main Body Systems: Glandular, hepatic, nervous

Physical: Asthma, bronchitis, coughs, digestive discomfort, liver support, pain relief, PMS, respiratory catarrh, skin concerns (mature, dry, wrinkles, fine lines), throat issues and urinary irritation.

Mental: Anxiety, confusion, indecisive, dizziness, exhaustion, fatigue, forgetful, hangover, headaches, hysteria, insomnia, mental strength, migraines, nervous, neurotic behavior, stress and tension.

Emotional: Anger, comforts the heart, emotional stuckness, grief, feel defeated, love of self and others, melancholy, modesty, obsessive, shy and not speaking up for self, suppressed and traumatic memories.

Chakra: 2nd (sacral), 4th (heart), 5th (throat), 6th (third eye), 7th (crown)

History: Both the ancient Greeks and Romans considered the violet to be a symbol of love. The Persians used the flowers to prepare sherbet. In medieval times, they were used to flavor Mead and other alcoholic drinks as well as added to culinary dishes. The violet seeds are loved by ants as food, and the plant attracts butterflies and other insects.

Personal Experience: I love this essential oil in my antioxidant facial toner, and to calm skin irritations and respiratory issues. It is a beautiful scent to quiet the mind, promote feelings of beauty and contentment, and reminds me that "I am enough".

Contraindications: Non-irritating.

Wintergreen *(Gaultheria procumbens)*

Scent: Camphoraceous, sharp, sweet with spicy undertones

Note: Middle to Base 7-8

Extraction Method: Steam Distillation

Part Used: Leaves

Plant Description: It is a low-lying, perennial evergreen shrub that can grow up to six inches high. It has dark green, oblong, shiny, hardy leaves with small, bell-shaped white-pink flowers and red berries. It prefers dry, acidic soil in shade to semi-shade with a little midday sunlight. It is drought tolerant. It is a member of the Ericaceae family.

Properties: Analgesic, antibacterial, anti-inflammatory, anti-rheumatic, antispasmodic, astringent, carminative, diuretic, decongestant, emmenagogue, expectorant, hepatotoxic, nervine, stimulant, tonic and vulnerary.

Chemistry: Esters (methyl salicylate); Carboxylic Acids (salicylic acid); Monoterpenes (pinene, myrcene, carene, limonene, gaultherilene).

Main Body Systems: Nervous, respiratory, structural

Physical: Arthritis, bee stings, bloating, cellulitis, circulation, cramps, digestive upset, fever, gas, intestinal spasms, joint pain, muscle aches, nausea, neuropathy, pain relief, respiratory and sinus congestion, sciatica, skin wounds, sprains, stiff neck and toothaches.

Mental: Alertness, concentration, confusion, creativity, indecisive, depression, determination, focus, headache, holds breath when stressed, invigorating, lifts spirits, and stamina, migraine, panic, refreshing and restores clarity.

Emotional: Anger, anguish, deep emotional wounds, discouraged, emotional stuckness, fear, feels deserted and alone, guilt, hopeless, loneliness, overcome negativity, strength to weather the storm, suppressed and withdrawn.

Chakra: 1st (root), 3rd (solar plexus), 5th (throat), 6th (third eye)

History: The genus was named for Dr. Gaultier, a Canadian physician of the mid-18th century. An extract has long been used to flavor teas, candy, medicines and chewing gum. Native American tribes used for aches and pains and to help breathing while hunting or carrying heavy loads.

Personal Experience: I love this essential oil to calm nerve and muscle pain, TMJ and open up respiratory passageways. Emotionally it brings clarity to situations and helps with decision making and alertness.

Contraindications: Can be toxic in large doses. Do not use internally. Avoid with aspirin allergies (contains methyl salicylate), asthma, epilepsy and during pregnancy.

Yarrow (*Achillea millefolium*)

Scent: Pungent yet slightly sweet, herbaceous, green with a slight camphor and floral undertones

Note: Middle 7

Extraction Method: Steam Distillation

Part Used: Flower

Plant Description: It is a rhizome spreading, perennial plant that can grow up to three feet tall. It has dark green, feathery fern-like leaves with clusters of small white or pink flowers. It can grow in poor, moist but well-drained soil in sunny climates. It is drought and frost tolerant. It is a member of the Compositae family.

Properties: Antibacterial, anti-inflammatory, antispasmodic, antiviral, astringent, carminative, cholagogue, cicatrisant, diaphoretic, emmenagogue, expectorant, febrifuge, hypotensive, insecticide, styptic, tonic, vasodilative and vulnerary.

Chemistry: Monoterpenes (sabinene, pinene, camphene, terpinene); Sesquiterpenes (chamazulene, germacrene, caryophyllene, humulene); Ketones (camphor, isoartemesia ketone, thujone); Monoterpenols (borneol, terpin-4-ol); Oxides (1,8 cineole); Esters (bornyl acetate); Lactones (achillin); and Sesquiterpenols (cadinol).

Main Body Systems: Circulatory, glandular, structural

Physical: Adrenal exhaustion, blood issues (internal and external bleeding, blood pressure, gums, nosebleeds), colds, cramping, hemorrhoids, PMS, poor circulation, skin concerns (scars, pigmentation, inflammation, acne [unclog pores], redness, eczema), urinary issues and vein health.

Mental: Calm chaos, concentration, confusion, indecisive, depression, fatigue, headache, insomnia, inner growth, intuition, mental stability, nervousness, relaxation, spiritually drained, self-confidence, stress and worry.

Emotional: Anger, anguish, bleeding or broken heart, constantly sacrificing self, deep emotional wounds, despair, grief, overwhelmed, protection from negativity and co-dependence, rejection, resentment, self-love, self-worth, taking on other's burdens and trauma.

Chakra: 1st (root), 3rd (solar plexus), 4th (heart), 6th (third eye), 7th (crown)

History: In 15th century, extensively used for headaches, nosebleeds, toothaches and wounds. Achillea originates from Achilles, legendary Greek warrior who made an ointment from the leaves for battle wounds during siege of Troy. A popular battle wound healing for many ancient cultures, it has been commonly referred to as soldier's woundwort or military herb.

Personal Experience: I love this essential oil for female concerns, anemia, cramps and wounds. Emotionally it grounds me and allows me to help people without taking on their burdens or negativity (especially when wearing hematite).

Contraindications: Use with a carrier especially with sensitive skin.

Ylang Ylang, *Canaga odorata*

Scent: Floral, heavy, powdery with sweet, balsamic and earthy undertones

Note: Middle 6-7

Extraction Method: Steam Distillation

Part Used: Flowers

Plant Description: It is a fragrant, tropical tree that can grow up to 75 feet tall. It has medium green, oval pointed leaves with drooping yellow (sometimes pink) flowers. It prefers moist, acid soil in warm, humid and sunny areas. It is frost sensitive. It is a member of the Annonaceae family.

Properties: Analgesic, antibacterial, antifungal, antidepressant, anti-inflammatory, antispasmodic, antiviral, aphrodisiac, cardiotonic, febrifuge, sedative and tonic.

Chemistry: Sesquiterpenes (caryophyllene, germacrene, farnesene, cadinene); Esters (benzyl acetate, benzyl benzoate, geranyl acetate, methyl salicylate, methyl benzoate); Monoterpenols (linalool); Ethers (paracresyl methyl ether); Phenols (methyl paracresol); Oxides (caryophyllene oxide); and Sesquiterpenols.

Main Body Systems: Circulatory, glandular, nervous

Physical: Adrenal exhaustion, alopecia, balance metabolism, calms blood pressure and palpitations, colic, heart tonic, hormone issues (PMS, hot flashes), liver support, rapid breathing, skin sebum balance and urinary concerns.

Mental: Anxiety, apprehension, contentment, dual personality, fainting, frigidity, hysteria, insomnia, mental strength, occipital headache, overactive mind, panic, restless, self-confidence, shock, stress, uplifting yet grounding and worry.

Emotional: Agitation, anger, bitterness, encourage self-acceptance, fear, grief, inner beauty, mend a broken heart, neglects own needs, obsessive, quarrelsome, repression, resentment, self-love, strengthens personal power, undernourished and trauma.

Chakra: 1st (root), 2nd (sacral), 4th (heart), 6th (third eye)

History: The name *ylang* translated by some as "flower of flowers". In Indonesia, petals were often strewn across the bed after marriage as a symbol of love. Used widely for perfumes. Major ingredient in Chanel No. 5. There are five grades based on time of distillation. Extra, which is the first distillation, most concentrated, strongest scent and finest oil. Next is Grade "1" which is distilled a second time from the same flowers within two hours. Followed by Grade "2" which is distilled within three to four hours; Grade "3" distilled up to fourteen plus hours. Ylang Complete is combination of all distillation stages.

Personal Experience: I love this essential oil to calm the heart on a physical and emotional level. It has helped female concerns, skin issues and glandular nourishment. Emotionally it helps one feel worthy, especially when sacrificing one's own needs for another.

Contraindications: Use caution with those with extreme low blood pressure.

Yuzu (*Citrus junos*)

Scent: Citrus, herbaceous and clean scent with floral, camphor and spicy undertones

Note: Top 2-3

Extraction Method: Cold expression

Part Used: Fruit rind

Plant Description: It is a fruit producing tree with a rounded top that can grow to heights of 25 feet. It has vibrant green, smooth, glossy leaves with round, white, star-like flowers and light orange round fruit with an irregular and bumpy exterior. It prefers hydrated but well-drained soil in warmer climates. It is frost tolerate but not drought tolerant. It is a member of the Rutaceae family.

Properties: Analgesic, antibacterial, antifungal, anti-inflammatory, antioxidant, antispasmodic, antiviral, carminative, immune modulator, nervine, sedative and tonic.

Chemistry: Monoterpenes (limonene, terpinene, phellandrene, myrcene, pinene); Monoterpenols (linalool); Ketones (yuzunone); and Sesquiterpenes (farnesene, caryophyllene).

Main Body Systems: Digestion, nervous, structural

Physical: Adrenal fatigue, arthritis, carbohydrate metabolism, cholesterol issues, cold and flu, digestive aid, enhance circulation, GI upset, gut clarity, immune (colds, flu), muscle pain and recovery, nerve relaxant, neuropathy, reduces endocrine stress, rheumatism, skin health and ulcers.

Mental: Anxiety, "calm, cool and collected", confusion, creativity, dementia, depression, insomnia, mental clarity, mood stability, negativity, nervous tension, panic attacks, PTSD, relaxation and worry *(http://www.ncbi.nlm.nih.gov/pmc/articles/PMC4048973/)*.

Emotional: Anger, centering, connect to inner strength, deprivation, emotional exhaustion, feel nurtured, forgiveness, frustration, hostility, inner strength, joy, regret, release emotional baggage, self-love, self-worth and soothes the soul.

Chakra: 3rd (solar plexus), 4th (heart), 6th (third eye)

History: One of the most popular citrus fruits in Japan and included in many culinary dishes, vinegars, beers and desserts. Contains a good amount of Vitamin C. The fruits are commonly added to bath water to enhance skin health, immunity and to promote overall well-being. An ancient hybrid of mandarin and papeda, first introduced to Japan during the Tang Dynasty for medicinal and nutritional purposes. It became more popular in the Unites States in early 2000's.

Personal Experience: I use this essential oil to relax the nerves, quiet the mind from excessive worry and to help recovery after times of physical, mental and emotional stress. It boosts my immune system and alleviates nerve pain.

Contraindications: Photosensitive.

Carriers & Bases

Carriers and bases are vehicles to transport essential oils into the skin when they cannot be used neat (applied directly to the skin). Examples are oils of almond, apricot and grapeseed. These are fat soluble and a great source for moisture, hydration and nourishment to the skin.

Carrier Oil Storage

Ideally carrier oils should be kept in the refrigerator or stored in a cool, dark area to prolong their shelf life. Many of the carrier oils have a six to nine month life span before turning rancid and begin losing their therapeutic value. Avoid direct sunlight exposure, high humidity and temperatures above 72°F as these can also destroy the therapeutic properties of these oils.

Labeling and Ingredients

Reading label ingredients can help to identify an oil's purity and benefits. It should list the botanical name to ensure property value. Listing ingredients with botanicals names is important if you are making your own products for this same reason. For example, avoid products that contain mineral oil as this creates a barrier on the skin making it hard to penetrate and absorb into the skin. Use caution with nut oils as some people have allergies to them. Olive oil is a great choice as long as it is extra virgin and cold pressed.

Activated Charcoal

Attracts, absorbs (like a sponge) and adsorbs (attracts like a magnet) toxins to help the body eliminate them. Most popular to combat food poisoning and over toxicity. Also has a drawing action on unwanted skin concerns. You can take the capsules internally and/or add to water, as well as apply topically in facial masks and skin concerns (i.e. warts, ringworm).

Almond (Sweet) Oil (*Prunus amygdalus, P. dulcis*)

Obtained from the nut of the almond tree, native to Asia and the Mediterranean. It is light to medium weight, non-greasy and absorbs easily into the skin. Expeller-pressed and provides moisture and hydration to all skin types. Shelf life is approximately six to eight months.

Aloe Vera Gel or Juice (*Aloe barbadensis*)

Light, cool, refreshing and healing to the skin. It is widely used for cuts, burns, sunburns, inflamed skin and wound healing. It offers hydration, nourishment and moisture to the skin. A natural preservative and has a shelf life of twelve months.

Apricot Kernel Oil (*Armeniaca vulgaris, Prunis armeniaca*)

A nut oil native to Asia, very fine and light weight. It provides hydration, soothes dry, damaged and mature skin and is high in vitamin A and B which help in cellular repair and rejuvenation. Shelf life is approximately six to eight months.

Apple Cider Vinegar

Ancient remedy for physical health ailments, hygiene, skin and mouth wash. Hippocrates used vinegar to manage wounds. It has also been employed for thousands of years for stomach ailments, skin irritations, sore throats, hair rinses and deodorants. It is antibacterial, antioxidant and removes dead skin cells with its powerful alpha hydroxy acids. Great as a toner, astringent or face wash for pH balance, acne and skin issues.

Argan Oil (*Argania spinosa L*)
Produced from the nut kernels of the argan tree, indigenous to Algeria and Morocco. Known to strengthen, hydrate and fortify skin, hair and nails. It is a medium weight oil, high in vitamin E and unsaturated fatty acids for intense moisture. Shelf life is approximately two years.

Arnica Cream or Oil *(Arnica montana)*
Obtained from flowers infused usually with olive oil, rich in essential fatty acids. It is a medium weight, yellow oil known for its anti-inflammatory, analgesic, antispasmodic and antibacterial properties. It has long been revered for its wound and bruise healing ability, pain relief and provides deep moisture and hydration to the skin. Shelf life is approximately twelve to eighteen months.

Avocado Oil *(Persea americana)*
It is a heavier oil made from the large seed in the center of the avocado fruit. It has a deep green color and rich in vitamin E, nutrients and monosaturated fats. Great for dry scalp, damaged hair, skin problems (eczema), dehydration as it absorbs easily into the skin. Keep in the fridge as it generally has a short shelf life of three to four months.

Baking Soda (*Sodium bicarbonate*)
An old and economical remedy used to cool, deodorize and cleanse. It absorbs perspiration and odors. Commonly used to clean surfaces, carpet, drains, toilets and to make body powders.

Black Ointment
It is known to be a drawing salve composed of several herbs such as chaparral, chickweed, comfrey, lobelia and plantain among others. Used to evacuate splinters, warts, cysts and debris in addition to combating bacteria, infectious wounds, ulcerations and hemorrhoids.

Calendula Cream or Oil *(Calendula officinalis)*
Commonly referred to as marigold, it is known for its analgesic, anti-inflammatory, antispasmodic, vulnerary and tonic properties. Derived from an infusion of the flowers, it heals burns, skin irritations, dry, chapped skin, rosacea (via strengthens blood vessels), swelling, edema and puffy eyes. For all skin types. Shelf life is approximately twelve to eighteen months.

Castile Soap
Originated in the Castile region of Spain, simply means that it is made from vegetable oil versus animal fat. A natural cleanser good for skin, pet coats and anything else that needs cleaning. It is properly pH balanced and offers great benefits to the skin. May leave a thin residue and greasy feel on hair. Shelf life is approximately three years.

Castor Oil (*Ricunus communis*)
It is expeller-pressed at a low temperature from the seeds of the castor oil plant. It is a heavier oil that offers protective qualities and seals in moisture and hydration. Historically used to reduce or minimize fibroids, cysts, acne and skin irritations as it is rich in essential fatty acids and is antifungal, antibacterial, antioxidant and anti-inflammatory. Shelf life is approximately twelve months.

Coconut Oil *(Cocos Nicifera)*
A semi-thick oil from the nut of the coconut palm tree, full of nutrients and essential fatty acids. Great to nourish, hydrate and moisturize skin, hair and nails, remove make-up and calm acne. Extra virgin and/or unfractionated coconut oil is the best to achieve therapeutic benefits for skin care. Fractionated or refined are other options, however they have a heavier molecular structure, but less of a coconut scent. It provides anti-inflammatory, antioxidant, antibacterial, antifungal and antiviral properties. Shelf life is approximately twelve to eighteen months.

Distress or Rescue Remedy
A combination of flower essences to help during times of crisis, panic, shock, trauma, anxiety and stress. Helpful before public speaking or entering into an uncomfortable or stressful situation. Physically, it aids in tissue, wound, muscle and joint repair, reduces swelling, calms itching, redness and inflammation. The Rescue Remedy is in a base of alcohol, while the Distress Remedy is in a base of glycerin so safer for children, and those with alcohol dependency issues.

Enzymes (Plant), Liquid
Plant enzymes break down protein structures such as insect exoskeletons, skin and pet dander, bacteria, germs and allergens. It also provides deep hydration of skin and tissues, driving nutrients deep within each layer of skin for optimal absorption. Shelf life is approximately two years.

Evening Primrose Oil (*Centhera biennis*)
A light to medium weight oil, high in GLA (gamma-linoleic acid), vitamins, minerals and antioxidants. It helps combat dry, devitalized, aging skin and calms skin irritations, scars and pigmentation. Shelf life is approximately eight months.

Golden Salve
This salve or ointment has antiseptic and vulnerary properties, helping with wound healing, cuts, burns, bruises, yeast infections, diaper rash and cold sores. It typically contains a combination of botanicals such as comfrey, chickweed, goldenseal, yarrow, marshmallow and mullein. Not recommended to use inside   of deep lacerations. Shelf life is approximately two years.

Grapeseed Oil *(Vitis vinifera)*
It is a fine, light, non-greasy and fast-absorbing oil that is hypo-allergenic and baby-friendly. It is produced from the grape seed, and for skin that does not absorb other oils very quickly. I find it to have a shorter shelf life of approximately three to four months, so don't let this one sit for a long time.

Green Tea (*Camellia sinensis*)
It is wonderful when added to a mist for its high in antioxidant and bioflavinoid, called catechins (anti-inflammatory), properties. It helps repair environmental and sun damaged skin and pigmentation. I make it up fresh from tea bags and distilled water.

Hazelnut Oil (*Corylus avellana*)
It is light weight made from the hazelnut kernel's oil, with a pleasant aroma and rich in vitamins, minerals and protein. It easily absorbs into the skin, astringent properties, some sun protection. Shelf life is approximately five to seven months.

Hemp Oil (*Cannabis sativa*)
It is cold-pressed from the hemp seed, and offers a good balance of antioxidants and essential fatty acids (omega 3 and 6) among other nutrients. It is a medium weight oil, with a molecular structure that resembles the body's, assisting in easy absorption. It provides immediate nourishment to the skin, tightens and tones elasticity and combats environmental and sun damage. Shelf life is approximately eight to ten months.

Honey (locally grown is best)
This is very thick, and sticky, but a great emollient, moisturizing and nourishing skin, nails and scalp. It helps remove impurities, heal blemishes and leaves skin glowing. Not recommended for children under three tears-old as it may clog their pores. Shelf life is approximately two years.

Hydrated Bentonite Clay
Derived from volcanic ash, it is full of nutrients and minerals. It is an absorbent (sponge) and adsorbent (magnet) for toxins, impurities, heavy metals and other internal contaminants. Great to use as a mask, after a little facial steam to nourish and hydrate skin, while removing debris and dead skin cells. Shelf life is approximately two years.

Jojoba Oil (*Simmondsia sinensis, Buxux sinensis*)
This is a liquid wax, not an actual oil. It is pressed and filtered from the bean-like seeds of the jojoba plant, providing moisture and hydration to the skin. It can balance dry and oily skin patches, nourish dry scalp and hair, skin irritations (eczema) and unhealthy cuticles. Shelf life is approximately two years.

Kukui Nut Oil (*Aleurites moluccana*)
A non-greasy oil, pressed from the seeds and historically known for its soothing and rejuvenating effects on the skin. It has the ability to penetrate quickly through the deepest layers of the skin, offering essential fatty acids, antioxidants and vitamins A, C and E to protect from the effects of aging, and nourish skin, scalp and cuticles. Great for all skin types. Shelf life is approximately one year.

Magnesium sulfate (Epsom salt)
A popular item in most households, it is historically known to detoxify the skin by drawing out toxins and impurities, while stimulating circulation. It helps alleviate sore muscles, upset stomach and constipation. Mix your essential oils in this to

emulsify before adding you're your bath or for a compress. Epsom salt with sea salt (equal parts) help soften hard water.

MSM Cream
MSM is known to help relieve pain, arthritis and oxidative stress. It repairs, strengthens and supports muscles, joints, tendons, ligaments and cartilage. Reduces stiffness and drives essential oils and herbal extracts deeper into tissues and muscles. Works especially well on pain and inflammation when combines with a glucosamine cream.

Neem Seed Oil (*Azadirachta indica*)
Scientifically shown to offer antibacterial, antiviral, antiseptic, antifungal, immune boosting, insecticide and vulnerary properties. NOT for ingestion.

Nigella sativa
Commonly refered to as black cumin seed is known for its analgesic, antimicrobial, anti-inflammatory, antihypertensive and antispasmodic properties *(http://www.ncbi.nlm.nih.gov/pmc/articles/PMC3642442/)*. It is a medium weight oil, high in vitmins A, B and C and has a slight nutty, pungent scent. It is beneficial for skin irritations, muscle soreness and fatigue. Shelf life is approximately two years.

Olive Oil (*Olea europaea*)
This is expeller-pressed from the olive fruit. It is a semi-heavy oil that provides hydrating, nourishing and moisturizing benefits. The highest quality is Extra Virgin, which is from the first pressing, and has the most vitamins and nutrients. The second pressing produces "classico" or "virgin" oil. Shelf life is approximately twelve to fifteen months.

Pau D' Arco Lotion
An antifungal, antiviral and antibacterial lotion that contains pau d'arco extract. Great to combat athlete's foot, candida, yeast infections, skin irritations, viral infections and digestive issues.

Progesterone Cream
Progesterone cream is a steroid hormone that can balances estrogen dominance, aids in overall hormone balance, relieves pain, aids in fertility, strengthens bones and combats vaginal dryness. It is a natural cortisone thus effective for relieving osteoporosis, arthritis, tendonitis and other inflammation.

Rosehip Oil *(R. rubiginosa)*
It is a light weight oil that is expeller-pressed from the fruit. It contains high amounts of rich essential fatty acids and vitamin C, which help with wound healing, hyperpigmentation (i.e. pregnancy mask) and damaged skin. It is beneficial for hormone concerns, to combat scar tissue and severe skin irritations. Shelf life is approximately six to eight months.

Safflower Oil (*carthamus tinctorius*)
This is a light to medium weight oil in the sunflower family, and known as the American saffron. It is extracted from the seeds and is best stored in the

refrigerator. It is high in unsaturated fats making it good for soft, supple, normal to dry skin. It contains Vitamin E, flavinoids, polysaccharides, arachnid acid and linoleic acid to reduce scar tissue, heal pigmentation and offer hydration. Shelf life is approximately nine to twelve months.

Sea Salts
These are very mineralizing to the skin, offering nourishment, removing toxin and dead skin cells, allowing for new skin cells to flourish. Great to mix your essential oils and botanicals in before adding to bath water, foot soak or compress. It should be obtained from an environmentally safe and reputable location.

Shea Butter *(Vitellaria paradoxa)*
This is a soft but thick wax made from nuts of the Shea nut tree in South Africa. It is rich in essential fats and vitamin E, providing antioxidant and skin healing benefits. It offers deep, long-lasting hydration and moisture to skin, and is mildly greasy on the skin. It is often used to nourish and soothe the feet (dry, cracked), hands, scalp, cuticles and skin. Ancient Egyptians used it to protect the skin against sun damage. You can use as a deodorant base as well. Shelf life is approximately one to two years.

Silver, aqua-sol (gel or liquid)
A liquid containing microscopic particles of pure silver suspended in distilled water that offer antibacterial, antiviral and antifungal properties. It is strong germicide and has been shown effective against over 600 disease-causing organisms. It is a valuable ingredient for antimicrobial products and protects the skin against foreign invaders. Hydrosol silver does not contain casein as colloidal silver. Shelf life is approximately two years.

Sunflower Oil *(Helianthus annus)*
This is a light to medium weight oil extracted from the sunflower seeds. It is high in Vitamins A, D and E as well as, minerals of calcium, zinc, potassium and iron, making it good for soft, nourished, normal to dry skin. Shelf life is approximately twelve months.

Witch Hazel *(Hamamelis virginiana)*
This is a plant distillation of the leaves, twigs and bark that offers many medicinal properties such as antioxidant, astringent, tonic and vulnerary. It is commonly used to tighten pores, minimizes wrinkles and fine lines, calm inflammation and bruising. It can be somewhat drying so limit the frequency of use. You can add in aloe vera gel in equal parts to minimize the drying effect if needed. Shelf life is approximately twelve to fifteen months.

Vitamin E Oil: (**d**-alpha <u>not</u> **dl**-alpha with tocopherols and tocotreinols)
This is great for just about any skin type, especially mature, sun-damaged and sensitive skin. It is considered to be a natural preservative and can be used straight or in combination with other carrier oils. It offers moisture and nourishment to skin irritation, scars, skin trauma and hemorrhoids. Shelf life is approximately two years.

Application Methods

Essential oils can be applied in one of three ways – inhalation, topical and internal. There are instances where it will be more beneficial to use one form of application over another so you want to evaluate each situation on a case by case basis. Essential oils are best used topically and via inhalation. Ingestion should only be considered when working with a highly trained, professional Aromatherapist and for a short duration, as toxicity, organ and membrane irritation may occur. It is contraindicated with certain health problems and prescription medications. Understanding an essential oil's chemistry, as well as the anatomy and physiology of the body and current health concerns need to be considered.

With any application method, a few considerations need to be addressed when working with children, adults, elderly and pets. First, what is the purpose of the blend? Next, what is the duration and frequency aromatherapy blend needs to be used? What is the rate of absorption needed to get the desired results? How will the body metabolize and excrete the blend, and is their physiology strong enough to handle the elimination process? Someone with chronic kidney issues, may want to use a smaller dilution ratio and inhalation method for short periods of time, rather than a strong, essential oil intensive topical blend, as the kidneys are responsible for the excretory process.

Inhalation

Inhalation will produce the most immediate effect. The aromas enter into the nose or mouth and travel via the respiratory tract. It takes less than one second for a pure oil to enter the body and produce a response. One popular way to use oils are through a diffusion such as ultrasonic, soapstone, aromaball and car diffuser. You can add a few drops of oil to pine cones or potpourri to emanate scents. You can create a room spray with distilled water and essential oils. You can use a facial sauna, steam room, shower or steam some water in a pot, add a few essential oils and do some deep breathing to aid with respiratory and immune support. Simple wafting is another form of inhalation. Wafting means you hold the bottle of essential oil under your nose, without touching your nose to the orifice reducer to avoid contamination. You will move the bottle from side to side, allowing your nose to pick up the scent without overwhelming your nose, and giving it breath to show you its full layers. Wafting can stimulate saliva, enzyme production and appetite. There is a method called 'drafting', in which you will hold the bottle of essential oil directly under one nostril and take five to ten deep breaths, then move to the second nostril. This method is used to satiate the taste buds curbing appetite and cravings. Be aware that some health concerns may be aggravated by steam such as asthma and epilepsy.

When conducting Olfactory Sensory Testing® with animals, you want to limit the scent exposure and give frequent breaks between scents. Their olfactory systems are much more sensitive due to the number of receptors in their nasal cavity. Cats are very sensitive to scent so it should be diffused in small doses. A dog, horse and llama are less sensitive than cats, but more sensitive than humans. With horses, have them smell per nostril, as each nostril connects to the opposite side of the brain.

Inhalation is beneficial for everyone, from birth to death. It activates us to respond and react. It triggers memories, calms or energizes our mind, restores the body and disinfects our environment. Another potent benefit to inhalation is in training, especially with someone who is deaf and/or blind. You can use various scents to help someone locate specific areas in the house, to condition them to know when to step up or down, and to tell what time of day it is. I have used this application for humans and pets.

Topical or External: Lotion, Massage Oils and Sprays
Dermal, topical or external applications work into the blood stream within 3 minutes. This is why it is important to use natural and pure products on the skin. When you apply an essential oil directly on the skin, it is called neat. I only recommend using lavender neat on the skin as other oils may cause skin irritations. Some external applications would be a lotion, massage oil or body spray. The essential oils are taken up by the lymph system and help to relieve sluggish and stagnate lymph. Eucalyptus and thyme are two of the most quickly absorbed essential oils. Once you have applied your essential oils to the skin, they usually remain in the body for about 20-90 minutes before they are excreted via urine, sweat, skin and exhalation.

Some forms of topical applications include a lotion or oil base, beneficial in massage, reflexology and Craniosacral. This is great to enhance relaxation, deep breathing, stimulate circulation and increase cell regeneration and turnover. It is also a nice technique to use with small babies to increase the bond between parent and child.

Contraindications for topical use include phototoxicity, skin and mucus sensitivities and irritations. Phototoxicity or photosensitive mean the essential oil contains a certain chemistry, like furanocoumarins, that can cause skin pigmentation when exposed to sunlight or artificial light (tanning beds). Certain chemical components are more irritating to the skin than others, so it is a good practice to cross-reference this when you are blending several oils together. Undiluted use, or neat applications have been known to manifest skin irritations and sensitization. Skin irritations usually produce an immediate reaction such as skin redness, itching and blotchiness. Skin sensitization is a type of allergic reaction that can be immediate, and in some cases, takes a little longer to occur. Continuous exposure may result in itching, redness, blotchy and painful skin. It is not recommended to apply undiluted essential oils to sensitive areas and membranes such as the ear, nose, vaginal and rectum. Do not use essential oils in the eye, as this can cause organ damage and even blindness.

Bath
Taking an Epsom or sea salt bath is the most commonly used form of aromatherapy. Dilute your essential oil(s) in the Epsom or sea salts before applying them to the bath water. Remember, your essential oils are not water soluble, so you don't want to add drops of essential oil straight into the bath water. This will cause a clump of oil to affix itself to one part of the skin versus being dispersed evenly throughout the bath water. If you want to make a salt scrub, simply add a carrier oil or aloe vera gel. You can also combine your oils in

a soap concentrate for a bath and body wash or shampoo. This is a great way to promote relaxation, stimulate the lymphatic and circulatory systems and to relieve edema.

I like to take a "Dreaming Bath" that integrates visioning, dreaming, relaxation, meditation and bathing. Bathing is a time to get clean, but also think of the significance of washing away the day's worries, challenges and burdens, and allowing the mind and body to renew, refresh and restore, preparing you for the next day. While you take a bath, close your eyes and dream. Mediate and envision what you would look like, and feel like, and be like if there were no constraints, no consequences and no boundaries. Often times, this is a great way to release tension, let go of fears and free your mind, allowing you to be present, in full mind and body, in joy.

Compress
A hot or cold compress is another external application. To use this method, mix a few drops of essential oil in Epsom or sea salt to emulsify. Then add to hot or cold water. You can dip a cloth into the water solution, wring out the excess and apply to the affected area. For best results, cover the cloth with a thick towel to hold in the heat or cold. This works well for fevers, swelling, inflammation, sprains, spasms and pain. Apply the compress to the area for 15 minutes, remove for 15 minutes and apply again for another 15 minutes. It is best to repeat this process, two or three times daily for more effective results. This is not recommended for an open wound area.

Perfume
Perfume comes from the Latin word *per fumare* meaning "through smoke". The Egyptians, Greeks and Romans used aromatic smoke from the burning of herbs for healing ceremonies, to cleanse bad spirits and to heal ailments. Today, we have a much simpler and more efficient way of creating perfumes, and they are also more cost effective. Perfumes can serve as a deodorant, stress relief or headache relief as well as help you on an emotional, mental and spiritual level at the same time. You not only smell good, but you can attain therapeutic benefits as well. One tip of caution, if you are applying a citrus-rich perfume to your skin, avoid direct sunlight for a few hours as it may cause a photosensitive response.

Making your own perfume is not only fun, but therapeutic. There are several ways to make up an aromatherapy perfume – standard blending or note layering blending. Standard blending would follow basic formulation techniques, such as making a list of all of the essential oils and carriers you want to include in your perfume, formulating, and blending all of these ingredients at once. Note that layering blending would consist of making a list of all of the top notes you want to include in your blend, all of your middle notes and all of your base notes. You will blend each of these note categories separately (in individual bottles or vials), and then combine all three of the categories together, in one bottle, to make up the final product. This layering process gives deeper dimension and scent depth, and smells more professional.

Suppository

To make a suppository, mix your essential oils in a golden salve solution. This is great for yeast infections and hemorrhoids. You can also mix essential oils with liquid plant enzymes or distilled water and probiotics to create a douche. This will help fight infection and replace some friendly flora. Use caution with severe hemorrhoids or internal bleeding.

Internal and Oral

We will not be discussing ingestion of essential oils in this course. For this application method, a highly trained and educated Level I and II certified Aromatherapist or medical professional should be consulted, as everyone is different. Internal use can be beneficial in certain situations, when the proper training has been employed, with the right safety precautions and blending techniques. The internal mucosal membranes are very delicate and excretory systems need to be functioning. Improper use may cause severe internal issues, disturbances and concerns. Essential oils contain chemical constituents that provide a variety of responses, but in excess, can be irritating. They should be respected and used appropriately. Remember, with knowledge and education come significant responsibility. Also, you want to make sure you are not considered as practicing medicine without a license. Each state has strict laws. We will not discuss internal use during this course.

Mouthwash

A mouthwash is another effective application for using your essential oils. To create a mouthwash, simply combine a few drops of essential oil to coconut oil and let emulsify completely before using (at least 30 minutes). Coconut oil is a wonderful fat emulsifier and offers many benefits to oral hygiene and health. Add in liquid plant enzymes and/or water in equal parts to fill the remainder of your container and shake well. You want to use approximately 10 drops of essential oil for a 2 ounce mouthwash. A great solution for gum health, thrush, dry mouth, excessive saliva and gum disease.

Update: The US Dept. of Alcohol, Tobacco & Firearms (27 CFR PART 21) prohibits the use of vodka and other intoxicating spirits as an ingredient in body care products without a permit. The US Federal Bureau of Alcohol, Tobacco and Firearms forbids the resale of drinking or beverage alcohol in perfumes and related products, regardless of whether you add essential oils, absolutes or other scenting materials. Adding beverage alcohols, such as vodka, to perfumes and then selling them is against the law because it is considered serving alcohol. Permits are required to serve alcohol. In order to stay within the law, you must use the formulas specified by US ATF for cosmetic applications. Local liquor control rules may also apply to beverage alcohol use in cosmetics and perfumes. (www.ecfr.gov/cgi-bin/text-idx?c=ecfr&sid=232b492e5b0bb9ba2198b4a56f883d8b&rgn=div6&view=text&node=27:1.0.1.1.17.6&idno=27)

Art of Blending

The best advice I can give you when you start blending and creating your own formulas and products is to keep a notebook or journal by your side at all times. Write down every blend you formulate and create, including your thoughts, results and lessons learned. This will also allow you to properly and accurately duplicate an effective blend.

When you are creating a blend, you want to blend with the outcome in mind. There are several factors to consider before you start formulating such as odor note, classification, intensity, purpose, chemistry, application, skin integrity and the person you are blending for. For most of your blends, it will be an integration of these qualities that help you achieve a successful blend. The quality of your ingredients is also important if you are seeking health and therapeutic results. An adulterated oil contains a different molecular structure, altered chemistry, scent recognition, delivery and excretion within the body.

Every essential oil has several layers of scent that permeate. They possess a top, middle and/or base note. Some oils are strictly a top note such as the citrus oils and some oils may be in between two notes such as cinnamon, which is a middle to base note. Let's take an in depth look at how these three notes differ.

The top note is the most light and volatile. It will vaporize quickly and last less than thirty minutes. These oils are generally uplifting and stress reducing. The middle notes are more stable. These scents unfold in about one minute to three hours after application. These notes blend out a softer tone and generally soothe and balance the body. Base notes are the least volatile. They are fixatives and hold blends together longer. They are heavier, thicker, deeper scented, warm, and sensuous. These notes are generally relaxing and grounding.

Olfactory Sensory Testing™

I created a system that helps an aromatherapist and client choose the best essential oils to include in a custom blend, and also facilitates in the formulation process. By using this system, you can determine which scents a client responds to the best, which also helps you organize them by strength and purpose.

The process of Olfactory Sensory Testing™ is simple. First, you will choose 10-20 essential oils (singles or blends) for your client to smell. You can place them on the counter in no particular order. Next, you will begin by taking one at a time of the essential oil bottles. You will smell it first, then extend your arm to allow the client to smell it, using the draft system (moving the scent from side to side under your client's nose). You will smell the essential oil scent first so you can connect and become familiar with that scent. It will also strengthen the connection between you and your client. When you smell the scent first, refrain from making a face or comment, as to not influence your client's response. By you holding the essential oil bottle for the client, it allows them to relax, so they can fully focus on taking in the dynamics and full aroma of the scent they are smelling. When you smell the scent, you want to lead by example, showing the client how to take in a deep breath and inhale the scent, then turning your head to the side to exhale, as not to breathe directly on the bottle's orifice reducer top (avoids contamination).

When you are doing this, explain this procedure and why to the client, so you educate them on the process.

Next, after they take in a full breath of the scent, ask them to rate the scent on a scale of 1-10, 10 being the best (I love it) and 1 being the worst ("yuck, no way"). As the client ranks the scents, you will place them in an order of 10's to 6's. For me, if it ranks a 6 or higher, this means I would use it. If it is a 5 or below, I most likely will not include that in the blend, unless that particular oil is a "must have" to accomplish a purpose, then I'll add 1-2 drops. All of the essential oils that ranked a 10, I group together. Then, all of the 9's I group together, and so on. Using the 3-2-1 blending rule (described in the next paragraph), I create my formulation. All of the 10's would have 3 drops each; all of the 9's would have 2 drops each; and all of the 8's would have 1 drop each. Keep in mind, this is just an outline or guideline to follow. There may be times when you have to adjust to include more oil choices. Here is an example:

Essential Oil Scents		Formulations: 2oz. Spray (20-22 total drops)			
			Score	3-2-1 Rule	Drops/EO
Lavender	9				
Mandarin	10	Mandarin	10	3 drops x2	6 total drops
Ylang Ylang	4				
Frankincense	7	Lavender	9	2 drops x2	4 total drops
Pine	6	Cinnamon	9	2 drops x2	4 total drops
Lemon	8				
Peppermint	8	Lemon	8	1 drops x2	2 total drops
Cinnamon	9	Peppermint	8	1 drops x2	2 total drops
Geranium	8	Geranium	8	1 drops x2	2 total drops
Lemongrass	7				20 Total Drops

Using the 3-2-1 blending technique, to achieve 20 total drops, we had to double each group of oils. So if you double the group that matches the 3 drops each (all of the 10's), that would give you 6 drops each. Doubling the group that matches the 2 drops each (all of the 9's), that would give you 4 drops each. And so on.

Formulations

When in doubt on how to formulate, follow the 3-2-1 blending rule. I first learned about this guideline from Larissa Jones in her book, *Aromatherapy For Body, Mind & Spirit*. This technique teaches that when you are formulating, if you need a starting point, or can't figure out how many drops of each oil to include, then you can formulate using 3 drops of a top note to 2 drops of a middle note to 1 drop of a base note. An example is 3 drops of lemon, 2 drops of geranium and 1 drop of frankincense. You would then adjust the total number of drops depending on the size and purpose of your blend.

Determining the odor classifications of each essential oil you will be including in your formulation can prove valuable. If you are creating a blend for a client who describes wanting a blend that is floral, light and uplifting, you will want to include your flower oils, some fruit and uplifting scents such as peppermint. If your goal is to have an earthy and grounding blend, then the formula above would not be accurate. Rather using oils such as patchouli, sandalwood and frankincense would be better suited.

When blending essential oils, you want to also pay close attention to the odor or scent of the oils. Smell the intensity of each oil and look at their viscosity and color. If a scent is light, thin and airy, such as bergamot, you may need to use more of this oil to obtain a desired aroma. If you are using a strong, earthy oil such as frankincense, you may need to use only a couple of drops to reach a desired scent. For example, if you mix bergamot with frankincense, you may want to use a two to one ratio or add a few more drops of bergamot than frankincense.

What is the purpose of your blend? Consider the physical, mental, emotional and spiritual benefits you are seeking from this blend. Essential oils are multi-dimensional, meaning they offer numerous benefits, simultaneously. Helichrysum for example has been historically shown to combat scars, skin irritations and nerve pain, but it is also known to calm excess liver emotions such as anger and frustration, and promote mental clarity and decision making.

Other factors that you may want to include in your formulation process is reviewing the chemistry of each essential oil that you will be including in the blend for therapeutic property strength. Application method will help you decide on two factors, one being the bottle choice and two is the number of drops to include in a blend. Does your application require a glass or BPA-free plastic bottle or jar? What size? In regards to the total drops of essential oil to include, consider skin sensitivities when it comes to topical applications. Know the person you are blending for and their skin integrity. Is the person an infant, adult, elderly or a pet? Do they have hardy skin or is it sensitive, thin or frail? Do they have severe health conditions? Any allergies? Other sensitivities?

Additionally, you can integrate various modalities into your blend such as Traditional Chinese Medicine and Ayurveda medicine. This added layer can further deepen the emotional and spiritual benefits of a blend. All of these factors are tools you have to formulate the best possible blend. You may integrate all of them into one blend, or pick a few. That is the beauty of custom blends…they are custom. Merging science with art, and skill.

As you prepare to formulate and mix up your blend, decide how you will measure out your ingredients. Will you measure by the drop using the orifice reducer on the essential, pipette, dropper or by weight? I personally like to handcraft each individual blend, whether custom or a mass batch, using the "by the drop" method via the bottle's orifice reducer. As in nature and life, nothing is ever perfect. The imperfections often is what makes it perfect. So I use drops when blending versus weight. But you decide which philosophy works best for you. The weight method can be more accurate and precise, especially when duplicating a scent over and over. However for me, it is more impersonal and takes away from that nature connection, and continuous energy flow of plant to bottle, that I like to have when blending.

Now that you have created your formula, it's time to mix it up. Your application method will often times choose whether you use a bottle or jar. With liquid blends such as room and body sprays, I like to add in the emulsifying ingredient(s) first, if you are using any. This will allow the essential oil drops to marry into and emulsify before you add in the liquid such as water or liquid plant enzymes. Next, add in the essential oils to the bottle so they can get acquainted and start bonding and emulsifying. This will also allow you to alter or adjust a desired scent more easily. If an emulsifier is being used, and you are able, let the blend sit for about 24 hours before adding in the remaining liquid carrier. If you are custom blending for a client, or need the blend quickly, try and let it sit for at least 15 minutes before adding in the carrier. After you have combined the essential oils, add your carriers, mix or shake well. Label each blend immediately and create a recipe card to track and monitor your results.

When blending bath salts, lotions, serums and massage oils, I like to mix everything up in a big bowl if possible and then add into the bottle or jar using a funnel to avoid spillage or a glass measuring cup with a pouring spout. If that is not possible, I add in about 50% of the carrier(s), whether an oil, lotion or salt, followed by the essential oils then an additional 25% of the carrier. I cap it, mix or shake well to disperse the scent throughout the carrier and then add in the remaining carrier, mixing and shaking it again to complete the blend. Label each blend immediately and create a recipe card to track and monitor your results.

Dilution Ratios & Measurements

There are a variety of ways to measure and combine your aromatherapy ingredients. Most large aromatherapy companies, medical aromatherapists and scientists weigh their essential oils and carriers by the gram, cc, or milliliter versus by the drop. For example, 1cc equals 1 ml equals 20 drops. This method offers a more accurate and precise formula that can be easily duplicated in mass quantities.

A more simplistic and less technical way to measure your formula is to calculate the number of drops per essential oil that is used. This is my preferred method. It is simple, easy and has produced very effective results. This method entails tracking the number of drops added to your product. When doing this, you must consider the size of the orifice reducer top and the viscosity (thickness) of the oil. This is most important when you are creating and blending a specific scent for emotional concerns.

There are blending and dilution guidelines to follow when you are using essential oils. Dilution ratio is the proportion of essential oil to an amount of a base or carrier. The amount of essential oil needed will vary from product to product and will depend on the purpose of the blend, application method, potency (weak or strong) and therapeutic results desired.

If the purpose of a formula is generic, such as energizing, use a 1% to 2% dilution ratio. For a more specific purpose such as a local or area specific massage, use a 2% to 4% dilution ratio since the effects will be concentrated in one area.

DILUTION RATIO CHART			
Size	1%	2%	4%
.5oz, 1T, 15ml	3 drops	6 drops	12 drops
1oz., 2T, 30ml	5 drops	10 drops	20 drops
2oz., 4T, 60ml	10 drops	20 drops	40 drops
4oz., 8T, 120ml	20 drops	40 drops	60 drops

The application method can dictate dilution ratios. This is important because water bases and perfumes may require more essential oil whereas massage oils, bath salts, mouthwash, suppository and diffusers may require less oil.

Potency can also guide your dilution ratio. What strength of a scent is needed for the blend? A stronger scent may be required for a stress formula and a softer scent for a massage oil.

Choosing Essential Oils

When choosing which essential oils to include in a formula or blend, there are a few factors to consider.

- Who is the blend for? An adult, child, elder or animal?
- What is the purpose of the aromatherapy blend? What needs to be accomplished? What are the mental, emotional, physical, nutritional and environmental concerns?
- Which quality essential oils do you have on hand? You may need to refer to your reference notes to match your oils with your blend's purpose. Cross-reference properties, chemistry and desired scent.
- What essential oils does your client like or dislike? Conduct Olfactory Sensory Testing™ (OST). Refer to your scent classification chart.
- What application method will be used for this aromatherapy blend? This may depend on which method your customer will actually use.
- Which dilution ratio will you be using? Refer to the Dilution Ration Chart.

Once you have answered the above questions, and you have compiled your list of ingredients (essential oils, carriers and bottle size), you are ready to formulate the amounts of each ingredients before blending it up. Make sure you document each recipe, corresponding adjustments and track the results. Here is the method I follow. I write it up on an index card and keep a record in my computer.

Name of Blend:		
Application Method:		
Ingredients	**Amount / # of Drops**	**Cost per drop or ounce**
Essential oil #1		
Essential oil #2		
Essential oil #3		
Essential oil #4		
Essential oil #5		
Carrier # 1		
Carrier #2		
Bottle Size		
TOTAL	# of Drops	Total Cost

Body System Introduction

I first learned about the body systems from Steven Horne, Master Herbalist, Iridologist, Author and Founder of the Tree of Light Institute *(www.treelite.com)*. He is a gifted healer, writer, practitioner, educator and speaker. He taught me about my body, mind and emotions when I was first getting started into holistic health, and that it changed my life forever. At the time, I was very sick, and I learned about the body and mind, to personally heal myself. In doing this, I found a gift in sharing my journey and empowering others with that same inspiration.

When we talk about the body systems, it is important to know that the human body is one unit, made up of several "departments". Our entire being is comprised of your physical body, emotions, spirit and soul. The body systems do not work independently, but rather synergistically. When one system does not function optimally, another will compensate or fall behind. This added stress may lead to "symptoms" and ailments.

The disharmonies and ailments we experience have a physical side and emotional side. To achieve optimal healing, you need to work on both to get to the true root cause and rebuild yourself. In my experience, I find that we spend more time being concerned with the quality of our clothes, shoes, appearance, purse, sporting gear and technology, than we do on the quality of our health. Then expect a quick fix when it's broken. Well, health doesn't work that way. We didn't get that way over night, so it will take time to stop the problem from occurring, repair the damage and rebuild the structure. In natural health, the rule of thumb I follow is allow 90 days for healing, plus one month for every year you have had the issue.

Herrings law of natural healing states that we heal from the top down (head to toe), inside out (internal terrain to outward manifestations) and in the reverse order of symptoms. Think of your body as a barrel. Everything you have endured and experienced is like adding one pebble to your barrel (aka, your body). At some point, your barrel will flow over, creating a "mess", unless you empty your barrel. So the reverse order of symptoms means that you will revisit, acknowledge, correct and release ailments that you have experienced most recently, to when you were born. This is excavating your barrel, or cleansing your barrel. When you don't cleanse your barrel, you suppress symptoms, and block or clog your elimination channels. This creates a state of imbalance and disharmony within your body and body systems.

Our body is comprised of a conglomerate of cells that are the basic components of all living things. Healthy cells are necessary to maintain healthy function, requiring oxygen, nutrients, hydration, energy and waste removal. In harmony, everything is normal. In disharmony, imbalances occur causing symptoms.

Nutrient deficiencies can mean our eliminative organs are weaker, therefore toxins accumulate and inflammation sets in. When there is less oxygen and nutrients delivered to the cells, they suffocate and die, leading to disharmony and ailments.

Understanding the ABCD's

Steven Horne, MH, AHG, IIPA, developed a simple and effective approach to understanding and applying natural healing, for personal use and professional practice. He discusses the ABCD's of health - activation, build, cleanse and direct aids. I often refer to these as the ABC's – **A**romatherapy, **B**ody, **C**olon.

A stands for Activation. This is finding those sources which stimulate or spark energy within the body such as a positive attitude, deep breathing, food enzymes and most importantly, aromatherapy.

B stands for Build the body and mind. This means you supply your body and mind with the nutrients and nourishment it needs to function such as vitamins, minerals, greens, probiotics and energizing aromatics.

C stands for Cleanse the body, mind and soul. These are botanicals that open up normal channels of elimination to allow the body to excrete toxins, such as herbal cleanses, Epsom salt baths, foot baths and the Far Infrared Sauna. Mentally and emotionally it is beneficial to cleanse negative thoughts, grudges, regrets and mental clutter, to allow for positivity, inspiration and motivation to fuel your passions. Freeing the body of these burdens can heal the soul and help it return to its authentic self.

D stands for Direct Aids. These are remedies and scents that are matched up to work on specific physical, mental, emotional and soul imbalances. I use these for acute situations that need immediate attention and usually takes a short period of time to recover like a urinary tract infection from not going to the bathroom often enough, or wiping incorrectly. Some urinary issues are chronic so further investigation is needed to choose the right protocol. For chronic situations, the protocol will often change weekly or monthly, to work on the culprits from various angles.

Understanding how the body works, and why certain situations occur when there is break down is critical when seeking remedies. You want to be able to effectively match up remedies that give you multi-functional purpose, as there are a lot of crossover symptoms in health.

Circadian Rhythm

The circadian rhythm is an endogenous 24-hour clock that controls physical, mental and behavioral processes in humans, animals and nature. It is what helps us get a restful sleep at night and have energy during the day, as well as optimum organ function for digestion, absorption, assimilation, utilization and elimination. It adjusts to the local environment we are exposed to by numerous external cues such as light, dark, time zone, daily schedule and molecular changes. Any imbalance in this clock, may contribute to physical, mental and emotional disharmony.

The circadian rhythm was first recorded in Greek history around 4th century B.C.E. and in Chinese texts around the 13th century. More extensive research has been conducted over the years from the 18th century to date. This rhythmic system is very insightful in understanding physiological and psychological processes in addition to how and why imbalances occur. One suggestion to monitor your health assessment, is to keep a journal of when symptoms, discomforts and problems occur to help narrow down which remedies might be beneficial for overall wellness *(https://en.wikipedia.org/wiki/Circadian_rhythm)*.

CIRCADIAN RHYTHM TIME CHART

Detoxification	11p - 1a	Gall Bladder	Bitterness
	1a - 3a	Liver	Anger
	3a - 5a	Lungs	Grief
	5a - 7a	Large Intestines	Worry
	7a - 9a	Stomach	Nourishment
Movement / Waste Removal	9a - 11a	Spleen	Joy
	11a - 1p	Heart	Balance
	1p - 3p	Small Intestines	Control
	3p - 5p	Bladder	Resentment
	5p - 7p	Kidneys	Fear
	7p - 9p	Circulation	Love
	9p - 11pa	Triple Warmer	Function

www.JennScents.com

Your body does maintenance on most of your eliminative organs at night while you should be sleeping. During this time of rest, your body can clean up debris, wrap up all of the trash and get it ready to discard when you wake up, all while being uninterrupted. Your "2nd adrenaline" kicks in at 11pm to give the energy needed to complete all of these tasks. So it is best to be in bed and asleep by 10pm, to give your body time to quiet down and enter into the REM cycle.

Your eliminative organs consist of the gall bladder, liver, lungs, colon, lymph and kidneys (includes skin). All but the kidneys and lymph are maintained at night. Each organ has an emotional connection, so when imbalances occur during certain times of the day, you not only want to look at the organ function disharmony, but the associated emotion as well. For example, bitterness, annoyance and feeling disrespected is connected with the gall bladder. The liver is associated with anger, frustration and irritability. The liver is responsible for so many functions, that when something doesn't go according to plan, it disrupts everything causing havoc. The lungs are connected with grief, guilt and sorrow. If we don't release burdens (via the colon), it backs up into the second lines of defense which is the respiratory system. This is where deep grief and trauma can manifest. The large intestine is where we hold worry. We must release those toxic burdens (physical, mental, emotion and spiritual) to allow for proper absorption and elimination, via the stomach.

The daytime processes include the spleen, heart, small intestines, bladder, kidneys, circulation and triple warmer functions. The spleen also includes the pancreas, and is responsible for joy, happiness and the "sweetness" of life. The

189

heart is all about rhythm, balance and harmony. The small intestines are associated with being over-analytical, overthinking, reading too much into something and high mental chatter. The bladder is connected with feeling invaded and not being able to release the toxic situation. We hold the emotion of fear in the kidneys, thus you will see chronic kidney issues and bedwetting (fear of a male figure). Circulation includes the lymphatic system and reproductive organs (sex, intimacy), and is associated with feeling loved, broken-hearted, abandoned or rejected. And last, the triple warmer or body's thermostat is actually a regulating and functional system, rather than an organ. It includes the endocrine system (adrenal, thyroid) which gives way for the second wind to be activated. If these are exhausted, then that second wind may only be able to inspire the eliminative organs at half capacity, thus not getting optimal elimination and disposal of wastes. The triple warmer is made up of the thorax, or upper function that controls intake; the abdomen, or middle function, which controls transformation; and the pelvis, or lower function, which controls elimination. In Chinese medicine, they link these three heaters or burners to the head, heart, lungs and chest, or upper region; the stomach and spleen-pancreas, or middle region; and the abdominal region to below the navel, or lower region.

Digestive System
The digestive system is made up of the stomach, liver, pancreas and intestines. Together they process food into a form we can use and deliver nutrients to the blood. It further breaks down food that consist of fats, carbs and proteins, into simpler components to allow for utilization of the nutrients. Beneficial essential oils are peppermint, Roman chamomile, lavender and thyme to combat upset stomach, gas, bloating, indigestion, cramping and heartburn.

Intestinal System
The intestinal system is made up of the small intestine, large intestine and appendix. Over 90% of digestion and absorption takes place in small intestine. This system is responsible for assimilating nutrients and eliminating cellular and solid waste, undigested food and reabsorbs water and electrolytes making (bowel) material firmer. 80% of our immune system resides in our intestines and guards us against infection. Beneficial essential oils are Roman chamomile, lavender, clove and marjoram to aid in intestinal cramping, IBS, Crohn's, Leaky Gut, diarrhea, constipation and inflammation.

Circulatory System
The circulatory system is made up of heart, arteries and veins. This system is similar to the transportation system of our roadways. It provides all living cells and the cardiac muscle with oxygen and nutrients and takes away the cell's wastes. Beneficial essential oils are rosemary, thyme, ylang ylang, black pepper and grapefruit to help stimulate circulation and lymphatic function, allowing for better blood flow, blood pressure function, calm irregular heartbeats and palpitations, unclog blockages and reduce the storage of toxins.

Respiratory System
The respiratory system includes the lungs, sinuses and lymphatic system. It is a vital system, taking oxygen into the bloodstream and removing carbon dioxide

waste. Oxygenated cells allow nutrients to be "burned", providing the necessary energy for the cell to function. Harmful bacteria and diseases have been shown to not thrive in highly oxygenated environments. Beneficial essential oils are eucalyptus, lemon, ravinsara, frankincense and ammi visnaga to enhance oxygen flow, removal of carbon dioxide waste, sinus infections, asthma, runny nose, congestion, allergies and dry and hacking coughs.

Immune System
You can't point to any particular organ or set of tissues and say, "here's the immune system". It encompasses lymphatic fluid, lymph nodes, spleen, bone marrow and thymus gland. The immune system promotes optimal immune function by combating bacterial, viral and fungal infections, relieving stress and fatigue and other compromising ailments. Immunity is a function of all body systems as they try to maintain normal homeostasis in the body by distinguishing between what belongs in the body versus what does not belong. Beneficial essential oils are cinnamon, lemon, clove, frankincense and tea tree.

Urinary System
The urinary system is made up of the kidneys and bladder. They filter body fluid concentrations via the kidneys and flushes wastes and toxins out of the blood, including heavy metals. It also contributes to proper pH and electrolyte balance for more energy production. In Chinese medicine, the kidneys build bone. The skin is also referred to often as the third kidney. Beneficial essential oils are pine, juniper, frankincense, and lemon to aid in kidney function, relieve urinary (UTI) and bladder infections, water retention and weak kidneys.

Nervous System (NS)
The nervous system is made up of the brain, spinal cord and nerves. It is an internal communication system, relaying signals and controlling every function of the body (heartbeat, secrete hormones, motor function). It allows us to respond to a situation, helps with memory, concentration, anxiety, stress, depression and sleep. The brain is a central computer where the NS functions begin and end. Beneficial essential oils are citrus, lavender, patchouli, clary sage, sweet basil and neroli. They are sedative and relaxant, to help calm nerves, combat memory loss, poor concentration, stress, irritability, insomnia and hyperactivity.

Glandular System
The glandular system is made up of the pituitary, thyroid, thymus, adrenals, pancreas and reproductive organs. Its purpose is to balances hormones (PMS, menopause, mood swings), emotional distress, growth spurts, sexual identity, body temperature, reproductive troubles and diabetes. Beneficial essential oils are red mandarin, cinnamon, geranium, sandalwood, melissa and palmarosa.

Adrenals
Made up of the adrenal glands, which sit atop of the kidneys. It is our alert system, regulates fluid, assist in reproductive function and our "fight and flight" responses. It secretes adrenaline (epinephrine) which stimulates the heart to maintain normal blood pressure, stress and blood sugar levels, as well as

secretes hormones that regulate metabolism and sex hormones. Beneficial essential oils are orange, pine, *Tanacetum annuum*, geranium and ylang ylang.

Thyroid
The thyroid gland, located at the base of the front of the neck, burns fat, regulates metabolism and heavily influences growth. Imbalances may be weight issues, emotional distress, intellectual ability or physical vitality. Beneficial essential oils are myrrh, myrtle, melissa, celery seed, geranium and palmarosa.

Pancreas
The pancreas is located below the left side of the rib cage. It manufactures digestive enzymes and secretes insulin (a hormone that regulates the amount of glucose [sugar used for energy] in the blood), which regulates blood sugar levels. We need enough sugar in the blood to keep the brain functioning properly. Dementia has been called Type III diabetes *(http://www.ncbi.nlm.nih.gov/pmc/articles/ PMC2769828/)*. Type I diabetes is developed in childhood and is insulin dependent. Type II diabetes is insulin resistant and often due to being overweight. Other imbalances may be anxiety, panic attacks or dizziness. Beneficial essential oils are pink grapefruit, lemon, lavender, coriander, geranium and parsley.

Reproductive
This system is made up of the ovaries (female) and testes (male). For women, ovaries regulate the reproductive process through hormone secretions (estrogen, progesterone, etc.), which are responsible for pregnancy, elimination and hormone balance. Beneficial essential oils are geranium, clary sage, sandalwood, cinnamon, frankincense, cypress and jasmine. For men, the testes develop, manufacture and store spermatozoa, and produce testosterone, which controls physical and mental characteristics. The prostate requires zinc for optimal functioning, as well as heavy metal cleansing. Beneficial essential oils are ylang ylang, lavender, cinnamon, cilantro and rose.

Hepatic System
The hepatic system is made up of the liver and gall bladder, which are both located on the right side of the abdomen, beneath the rib cage. Their job is to assist in the nutrient assimilation, store nutrients and blood until they are needed, filter out and destroy toxins, eliminate excess cholesterol, combust hormones for use and many other important functions. Beneficial essential oils to stimulate a sluggish hepatic system are citrus, cypress, rosemary, ginger, basil and anise. Beneficial essential oils to calm and support and an overactive hepatic system are patchouli, helichrysum, mints, chamomiles, niaouli and rose.

Structural (Muscular and Skeletal) System
The structural system is made up of skin (largest eliminative organ), skeleton (bones), muscles, membranes and connective tissue. It provides support and structure for the body to protect vital organs (notably brain, spinal cord, heart and lungs), assist in movement and help produce blood cells. Beneficial essential oils are helichrysum, carrot, oregano, ginger and cypress to support skin, hair, nails and bones, arthritis, joint pain, osteoporosis, muscle cramps, poor posture, alopecia, scar tissue buildup and skin irritations.

192

Ethical Personal & Professional Guidelines

Ethics is an important part of business. It builds a foundation of trust and respect between you and your clients. There are several factors to consider when operating an ethical business - integrity, credibility, respect, morals and values, doing the right thing, consistency, responsibility and confidentiality. Let's look at each of these traits in greater detail.

Integrity of Yourself, Your Business, Your Reputation and Your Client

Integrity: (in teg' ri tē), noun. 1. uncompromising adherence to moral and ethical principles; soundness of moral character; honesty. 2. the state of being whole or entire: to preserve the integrity of an empire. 3. sound or unimpaired condition. - Syn. Honor *(Random House Webster's College Dictionary, Second Edition, 1997)*

Credibility: Be Honest and Fair

Credibility: (kredə' bilədē), noun. 1. the quality of being trusted and believed in. 2. The quality of being convincing or believable. 3. refers to the objective and subjective components of the believability of a source or message *(http://en.wikipedia.org/wiki/Credibility)*.

Respect

Treat your client like family. Obey and be mindful to their principles, morals, traditions, beliefs. Follow the golden rule, "Do unto others as you would have them do unto you". Luke: 6:31 Respect: (rə' spekt), noun. 1. a feeling of deep admiration for someone or something elicited by their abilities, qualities, or achievements. 2. a particular aspect, point, or detail. Verb. 1. admire deeply, as a result of their abilities, qualities, or achievements.

Morals & Values

Stay faithful to your belief, don't give in to influence and respect others' morals and values. Moral is an adjective defined as being concerned with the principles of right and wrong behavior and the goodness or badness of human character. As a noun it is defined as person's standards of behavior or beliefs concerning what is and is not acceptable for them to do. It is said to be the motivation for how we judge ourselves and others.

Values are the rules by which we make our decisions about right and wrong, good and bad, and guide our behavior. Morals and values are both part of the "ethics system" by which we conduct ourselves, personally and professionally.

Doing the Right Thing

Doing the right thing can sometimes be shadowed by influence and temptation. Some key points worth mentioning are Do NOT:
- Judge
- Discriminate
- Lie / dishonesty
- Steal / theft
- Provide misleading information or instructions
- Do something the client asked you not to do

Be Consistent
Provide consistent services, be on time (or early) consistently, discuss aromatherapy safety, details and instructions consistently and consistently share your disclaimer.

Responsibility
Aromatherapy must be used responsibly through the application of factual knowledge, professionalism and common and moral sense. If you are not sure of an answer or response, DO NOT guess. Be honest, do your research and completely understand a topic before discussing with others. With knowledge and business, comes responsibility.

Education
Educate yourself about essential oil safety, precautions, usage, properties, benefits and applications prior to using essential oils with a client, or teaching others. Practice with family and friends before offering aromatherapy to a client. It is highly recommended that you do not apply essential oils undiluted, directly to the skin without proper and extensive professional training and education. Understanding the body's anatomy and physiology is extremely important, as to do no harm, or give a false sense of comfort about a particular essential oil. Many undiluted essential oils may cause skin irritation and an unfavorable response, unless emulsified in a fat based carrier that can offer proper delivery, absorption and excretion by the body. Receptor sites can become blocked and irritated in some instances, so practicing proper safety measures based on your level of training is practicing ethical behavior.

Business education is equally important to make sure you are operating a healthy business. SCORE (Service Corps of Retired Executives) is a great resource to help you develop and grow your business. I call this organization "guidance counselors for businesses". They offer a variety of mentors to help you review strategies, industry resources and growth strategies. You can research more at www.SCORE.org.

Confidentiality
Keep the information shared between you and your client confidential and do NOT share these private details with anyone (including family members). Your client needs to know they can trust you. Privacy and discretion must be used when talking with a client, especially in public or to another person.

Client Files
Keep all client files in a safe and secure location. Do not allow anyone to go through your client files as this contains personal and confidential information.

Practice Aromatherapy Legally
It is in your best interest, personally and professionally to understand and follow your state and federal laws (as well as the guidelines set forth from the National Association of Holistic aromatherapy – www.NAHA.org) as they pertain to the industry of aromatherapy. NAHA has a free teleseminar available in their Bookstore on the Art of Languaging if you'd like to further educate yourself.

Professional Image & Hygiene

You only get one chance to make a first impression with a client and to keep them coming back. Maintenance of yourself is important, as you are a walking advertisement of yourself, your brand and your image. It is equally important for the sake of everyone's health, like brushing your teeth, combing your hair and wearing clean clothes that fit. Especially since you will be spending some time with your clients during the interview process and blending session.

Your appearance and grooming practices can secure a loyal customer, or shy them away. You want to look the part and smell the part, making your clients feel comfortable, invited, safe and secure. Ask yourself, what image do you want to portray to your clients? You can stay true to who you are and express your style in a professional manner.

Here are some do's and don'ts when it comes to personal appearance, presentation and hygiene.

- Do wear deodorant. When using a natural deodorant, it is helpful to reapply several times throughout the day. Liquid chlorophyll is a natural internal deodorizer, so adding some to your water daily can help with body odor. Perspiration doesn't actually smell. It is the toxins attached to it that smell. So if you are experiencing body odor, you may want to consider a cleanse or detox.
- Do wear clothes that fit. If your clothes are hanging down, too long or too tight, it can inhibit your movement, as well as affect your circulation.
- Do not wear synthetic perfumes and fragrances. Many people have allergies or are sensitive to the potency of strong, chemical based perfumes. Not to mention it distorts the sense of smell, which would be unfortunate during an aromatherapy session.
- Do not smoke prior to or during a meeting with a client. Smoking can affect the olfactory systems ability to smell and process scent.
- Do not wear dangling and loud jewelry, especially on the wrist when conducting Olfactory Sensory Testing™. The clanking of jewelry can be distracting when your client is trying to relax and take in a scent.
- Create an inviting, positive atmosphere, where your client can focus on connecting with the scents. Refrain from using negative language and creating a hostile environment.

When blending, it has been said to wear solid color clothing like black and white. Adding in this layer of color therapy can allow the essential oil molecules to flow freely, without distraction from loud and bold prints. Color has been shown to inspire mood, behavior, energy, emotions, responses and reactions, just as scents do. So combining color with scents can enhance your client's overall experience. You also want to be comfortable with what you are wearing when blending so you have mobility and flexibility.

A-Z Recipes for Everyday Health Concerns
For Women, Men, Children & Pets

My recipes include ingredients, blending instructions and directions for use. I use the essential oil common name, but yu can refer to the Essential Oil Profile section for their botanical names. If a particular species was used, it will be noted. These recipes are recommendations and substitutions can be made as needed. These are general guidelines and not intented to replace medical advice.

Aftershave

Distilled Water	1 ounce
Aloe Vera Gel	.50 ounces
Unscented Lotion	.50 ounces
Aqua-sol Silver	10 drops
Lavender	8 drops
Tea Tree	6 drops
Patchouli	2 drops

Instructions: In a 2 ounce bottle, add in the aloe vera gel followed by the essential oils. Swirl this around to emulsify the oils into the carrier. Next, add in the unscented lotion carrier and aqua-sol silver. Shake the bottle to immerse blend those ingredients together. Last, add the distilled water. Shake well until blended.

Directions for Use: Apply a dime size amount to dry skin using a small circular motion. It will leave skin feeling smooth and refreshing.

Adrenal Support Mist

Distilled Water	1 ounce
Liquid Plant Enzymes	1 ounce
Aqua-sol Silver	10 drops
Tanacetum annuum	8 drops
Red Mandarin	6 drops
Benzoin	6 drops

Instructions: In a 2 ounce bottle, combine the essential oils first. Follow with the aqua-sol silver, liquid plant enzymes and distilled water. Shake the bottle well to blend the ingredients together.

Directions for Use: Spray around you three to four times to rejuvenate the adrenals and combat exhaustion and fatigue.

Allergy Relief Spray

Liquid Plant Enzymes	2 ounces
Lavender	6 drops
Eucalyptus	5 drops
Frankincense	5 drops

Instructions: In a 2 ounce bottle, combine the essential oils first, followed by the liquid plant enzymes. Shake well.

Directions for Use: Spray three to four times around you to diminish allergens and to relieve allergy symptoms such as sneezing, runny nose, watery eyes and puffy skin. Use as often as needed.

Appetite Suppressant

Unscented Carrier Oil	.33 ounces
Bergamot	3 drops
Coriander	2 drops
Grapefruit, Pink	3 drops
Fennel	2 drops

Instructions: In a .33oz. roll-on bottle, add in half of the carrier oil, followed by the essential oils. Swirl around to mix them together, then add in the remaining unscented carrier oil. Shake well.

Directions for Use: Apply to wrist, neck, above the lip and throat area as needed to control appetite, food cravings and low blood sugar. To make a spray, substitute distilled water for the unscented carrier oil.

Arthritis Rub

Arnica and/or Calendula Cream	1 ounce
MSM Cream	.50 ounces
Aloe Vera Gel	1 ounce
Unscented Lotion	1.50 ounces
Lavender	6 drops
Chamomile, Roman	6 drops
Frankincense	5 drops
Marjoram	5 drops
Birch	4 drops
Cypress	4 drops

Instructions: In a 4 ounce jar, combine the Arnica and/or Calendula cream, MSM cream, aloe vera gel and all of the essential oils. Mix well. Next, add in the unscented lotion and blend well.

Directions for Use: Apply to affected area twice daily and as needed to calm pain and discomfort.

Baby Massage Lotion

Aloe Vera Gel or Unscented Lotion	2 ounces
Lavender	7 drops
Red Mandarin	4 drops
Chamomile, Roman	3 drops

Instructions: In a 2 ounce bottle, add 1 ounce carrier and all of the essential oils. Cap and shake well. Fill the remainder of the bottle with the rest of the carrier, cap and shake well until oils are completely blended into the carrier.

Directions for Use: Apply a small amount of lotion to the baby's skin in a circular motion. This will increase circulation and lymphatic system movement while creating a bond between you and child. Helpful to quiet a baby and promote a restful sleep.

Belly Rub (for stretchmarks and scars)

Unscented Lotion	1 ounce
Jojoba Oil	10 drops
Rosehip Oil	1 teaspoon
Vitamin E Oil	1 teaspoon
Shea Butter	.50 ounces
Lavender	10 drops
Red Mandarin	5 drops
Frankincense	3 drops
Helichrysum	3 drops

Instructions: In a 2 ounce jar, mix all of the carrier oils together with the essential oils. Mix well. Next, add the unscented lotion base and mix well.

Directions for Use: Apply generously in a circular motion to affected area. For best results, use two to three daily and as needed.

Bernie's Blend Bath Oil

Unscented Carrier Oil	2 ounces
Peppermint	5 drops
Lavender	5 drops
Marjoram	4 drops
Eucalyptus	4 drops
Pine	2 drops

Instructions: In a 2 ounce bottle, combine the essential oils and the unscented carrier oil. Shake well.

Directions for Use: Apply .5 - 1 ounce to running water. Sit back and relax as you relieve muscle aches and pains while rejuvenating the senses.

Broken Bones

Arnica and/or Calendula Cream	1.50 ounces
Golden Salve	1 ounces
MSM Cream	.50 ounces
Unscented Lotion	1 ounces
Chamomile, Roman	8 drops
Lavender	10 drops
Helichrysum	4 drops
Frankincense	4 drops
Thyme, Sweet	4 drops
Oregano	2 drops

Instructions: In a 4 ounce jar, mix the Arnica/Calendula cream, Golden Salve and MSM cream together, followed by the essential oils. Mix until it is smooth and chunk-free. Next, add the unscented lotion. Mix thoroughly.

Directions for Use: If possible, apply in a circular motion to and around the affected area four to six times daily. Wrap in a breathable gauze.

Circulation Lotion

Unscented Lotion	3 ounces
Aloe Vera Gel	1 ounce
Cypress	8 drops
Geranium	6 drops
Juniper	4 drops
Cinnamon	7 drops
Ginger	5 drops

Instructions: In a 4 ounce jar, add 2 ounces of the unscented lotion and 1 ounce of aloe vera gel, followed by the essential oils. Mix well. Next add in the remaining carrier lotion and mix well.

Directions for Use: Massage into skin using a small circular motion, twice daily.

Cold Sore Balm

Golden Salve	.50 ounces
Arnica and/or Calendula Cream	.25 ounces
Aloe Vera Gel	.25 ounces
Melissa	2 drops
Bergamot	3 drops
Lavender	2 drops
Ravinsara	2 drops

Instructions: In a 1 ounce jar, mix the golden salve and Arnica/Calendula Cream together until smooth. Next, add the essential oils and aloe vera gel. Mix well.

Directions for Use: Apply small amount to affected area three to four times daily and as needed for discomfort and pain.

Colic Relief

Aloe Vera Gel	.33 ounces
Chamomile, Roman	5 drops
Lavender	1 drop
Peppermint	1 drop

Instructions: In a .33 oz. roll-on bottle, mix the essential oils followed by the aloe vera gel. Shake well. If your aloe vera gel is thick, add in a little distilled water to thin it out so it does not clog the rollerball.

Directions for Use: Apply to abdomen and temples as needed for discomfort and irritability.

Concentration Spray (for focus and alertness)

Distilled Water	2 ounces
Rosemary	6 drops
Lemon	5 drops
Mandarin, Red	5 drops
Peppermint	4 drops

Instructions: In a 2 ounce bottle, mix the essential oils followed by the distilled water. Shake well.

Directions for Use: Spray around you when you need to focus and concentrate. For test taking, spray around you and breathe in while studying and again when you are retrieving the information at test time. Great for memory association and recall.

Cysts & Fibroids

Unscented Lotion	.75 ounces
MSM Cream	.25 ounces
Black Ointment	.50 ounces
Castor Oil	.50 ounces
Cypress	3 drops
Frankincense	3 drops
Thyme	3 drops
Helichrysum	2 drops
Lavender	5 drops

Instructions: In a 2 ounce jar, mix the black ointment, MSM cream and unscented lotion until it is smooth. Blend thoroughly until there are no more chunks. Add in the essential oils and castor oil. Mix well and shake before use.

Directions for Use: Apply to cystic area three to four times daily in a circular motion using the fingertips. Massage for about ten to fifteen minutes.

Deep Pain Relief Spray

Liquid Plant Enzymes	2 ounces
Clove	8 drops
Ginger	8 drops
Birch	3 drops
Frankincense	3 drops

Instructions: In a 2 ounce bottle, mix the essential oils and liquid plant enzymes. Shake well.

Directions for Use: Spray two to three times to affected area to relieve sore, tense, stiff and overworked muscles and joints. For best results, follow with the Sports Rub recipe listed in this book.

Diaper Rash Balm

Golden Salve	.50 ounces
Aloe Vera Gel	.50 ounces
Geranium	3 drops
Lavender	3 drops
Tea Tree	2 drops
Chamomile, Roman	2 drops

Instructions: In a 1 ounce jar, mix the golden salve and essential oils until blended and smooth. Next, add the aloe vera gel and mix thoroughly.

Directions for Use: Apply to affected area after each diaper change to relieve red, itching, inflamed, dry and chapped skin. Use as needed.

Earache (fluid build-up)

Unscented Carrier Oil	1 ounce
Helichrysum	6 drops
Marjoram	2 drops
Lavender	2 drops

Instructions: In a 1 ounce bottle with a dropper, combine the essential oils and carrier oil. Shake well.

Directions for Use: Apply 10-15 drops, four to six times daily to the outer ear area. Massage this area with your fingertips for about 10-20 minutes to stimulate circulation and release lymphatic congestion. For best results, you can warm up this oil by sitting it in some warm water, or rubbing your hands together to create heat, then adding some oil to your hands before applying to the ears.

Fear Away Spray

Distilled Water	2 ounces
Frankincense	6 drops
Pine	3 drops
Juniper	3 drops
Lemon	3 drops
Mandarin, Red	4 drops

Instructions: In a 2 ounce bottle, combine the essential oils and distilled water. Shake well.

Directions for Use: Spray around you 3-4 times when fearful, anxious, nervous or insecure. This blend will dispel feelings of fright, unknown fears and worry, fear of the unknown and feelings of being unsafe. Use as often as needed. For best results, add in 2-4 drops of Mimulus Bach Flower Remedy to the blend.

Fibromyalgia Serum

Unscented Carrier Oil	2 ounces
Ravinsara	6 drops
Lavender	5 drops
Helichrysum	2 drops
Pine	3 drops
Mandarin, red	3 drops

Instructions: In a 2 ounce bottle, add essential oils with carrier oil. Shake well.

Directions for Use: Apply to sore and weak muscles, areas of discomfort, spine and solar plexus. Use at least twice daily. Great to lift spirits and promote a positive attitude.

Flea Control

Liquid Plant Enzymes	4 ounces
Eucalyptus	4 drops
Lavender	6 drops
Thyme	4 drops
Tea Tree	3 drops
Rosemary	4 drops
Citronella	4 drops
Neem	4 drops

Instructions: In a 2 ounce bottle, mix essential oils and liquid plant enzymes. Shake well.

Directions for Use: Apply to flea stricken areas, surfaces and fabrics three times daily until problem dissipates. Massage into the skin of humans and coat of animals. Remember, fleas lay eggs so you want to use a second wave of sprays one to two weeks later. You can also spray a couple of times on a bandana and place around pet's neck.

Grief Relief Spray (and Respiratory Concerns)

Liquid Plant Enzymes	2 ounces
Distress or Rescue Flower Remedy	4 droppers
Ravinsara	8 drops
Bergamot	5 drops
Frankincense	2 drops
Rose	2 drops
Sandalwood	2 drops

Instructions: In a 2 ounce bottle, mix essential oils and the Distress or Rescue Remedy. Mix well. Next, add in the liquid plant enzymes. Shake well.

Directions for Use: Spray around you several times daily and as needed for grieving moments. Helps to relieve overwhelming feelings of grief, weepiness, despair, sorrow, chest tightness, a lump in the throat, fatigue, sinus congestion and exhaustion.

Hair Detangling Spray

Liquid Plant Enzymes	1.50 ounces
Aloe Vera Gel	.50 ounces
Chamomile, Roman	3 drops
Lavender	10 drops
Rosemary	5 drops

Instructions: In a 2 ounce bottle, mix the essential oils with the aloe vera gel. Mix well. Next, add in the liquid plant enzymes and shake well.

Directions for Use: Spray hair and massage mist into the tangled areas. Leave in for one to two minutes before brushing or combing hair.

Hand Sanitizer Spray

Liquid Plant Enzymes	1.75 ounces
Aqua-sol Silver	.25 ounces
Lavender	6 drops
Lemon	5 drops
Thyme	2 drops
Cinnamon	5 drops
Oregano	2 drops

Instructions: In a 2 ounce bottle, combine the essential oils with aqua-sol silver and liquid plant enzymes. Shake well.

Directions for Use: Spray on hands and rub together, or mist surfaces to disinfect and fight against germs, bacterial and viruses.

Hand Sanitizer Gel

Aloe Vera Gel	1.75 ounces
Liquid Plant Enzymes	.25 ounces
Tea Tree	5 drops
Thyme	5 drops
Lemon	5 drops
Clove	5 drops

Instructions: In a 2 ounce bottle, combine the essential oils with the aloe vera gel. Mix well. Next add in the liquid plant enzymes and shake well.

Directions for Use: Apply to hands and rub together, or apply to surfaces and wipe down to disinfect and fight against germs, bacterial and viruses. This formula stops the spread of infection. Thyme, lemon and clove were three oils used during the WWI to disinfect the hospitals. Ironically their initials are TLC.

Headache Roll-on

Unscented Carrier Oil	.33 ounces
Lavender	3 drops
Peppermint	6 drops
Rosemary	2 drops
Lemon	1 drop

Instructions: In a .33 ounce glass roll-on bottle, add in half of the carrier oil with the essential oils. Mix well, then add in the remaining carrier oil. Shake well.

Directions for Use: Apply as needed to temples, hairline and back of neck to relieve pain, tension, nausea and discomfort associated with headaches.

Hemorrhoid Salve

Golden Salve	.50 ounces
Aloe Vera Gel	.25 ounces
Unscented Lotion	.25 ounces
Yarrow	1 capsule
Lavender	2 drops
Chamomile, Roman	3 drops
Geranium	2 drops
Cypress	1 drop

Instructions: In a 1 ounce jar, combine the golden salve and aloe vera gel. Blend well. Mix in the yarrow capsule and essential oils followed by the unscented lotion and blend until smooth.

Directions for Use: Apply to affected area after each restroom visit, before bed and as needed for pain, discomfort and itch.

Hiatal Hernia

Unscented Carrier Oil	.33 ounces
Distress or Rescue Flower Remedy	5 drops
Chamomile, Roman	7 drops
Marjoram	1 drop
Lavender	2 drops

Instructions: Combine essential oils, Distress or Rescue Remedy and unscented carrier oil in a .33 ounce roll-on bottle. Shake well.

Directions for Use: Apply to chest to abdomen area. Using your middle and ring fingers, massage in a downward motion for approximately three to five minutes. This will help relieve the stomach from discomfort.

Horse Fly Repellent

Liquid Plant Enzymes	4 ounces
Neem	4 drops
Citronella	4 drops
Geranium	4 drops
Pine	4 drops
Peppermint	4 drops

Instructions: In a 4 ounce bottle, combine the essential oils and liquid plant enzymes. Shake well.

Directions for Use: Apply surrounding area around the horse several times a day, and as needed.

Hot Flash Spray

Liquid Plant Enzymes	2 ounces
Lavender	3 drops
Peppermint	3 drops
Lemongrass	2 drops
Geranium	4 drops
Clary Sage	4 drops
Chamomile, Roman	2 drops
Frankincense	2 drops

Instructions: Combine essential oils and liquid plant enzymes in a 2 ounce bottle. Shake well.

Directions for Use: Spray as needed for hot flashes and night sweats. Also, spray bed linens, pajamas and surroundings before bed to promote a more restful sleep. Take note if hot flashes present themselves during a stressful situation or certain time of day. If so, spray yourself about 15-20 minutes prior to the event.

Hydrating Facial Toner

Liquid Plant Enzymes	1.75 ounces
Aqua-sol Silver	.25 ounces
Lavender	7 drops
Chamomile, Roman	4 drops
Carrot Seed	3 drops
Helichrysum	2 drops

Instructions: In a 2 ounce bottle, combine essential oils, aqua-sol silver and liquid plant enzymes. Shake well.

Directions for Use: Apply twice daily to face, neck and chest to hydrate and nourish the skin. Encourages cell turnover, repair and rejuvenation.

Infertility Massage Oil (for women)

Unscented Carrier Oil	2 ounces
Bergamot	5 drops
Clary sage	4 drops
Geranium	4 drops
Helichrysum	3 drops
Chamomile, Roman	2 drops
Jasmine	1 drop

Instructions: In a 2 ounce bottle, combine essential oils and unscented carrier oil. Shake well.

Directions for Use: Apply to wrist, neck, ankle bones, inner thighs and lower abdomen area twice daily.

Infertility Massage Oil (for men)

Unscented Carrier Oil	2 ounces
Bergamot	4 drops
Clary sage	3 drops
Geranium	3 drops
Helichrysum	1 drop
Clove	4 drops
Cypress	2 drops

Instructions: In a 2 ounce bottle, combine essential oils and unscented carrier oil. Shake well.

Directions for Use: Apply to wrist, neck, ankle bones, lower abdomen, inner thighs and male reproductive area twice daily.

Insect Bite Relief Spray

Liquid Plant Enzymes	3.75 ounces
Aqua-sol Silver	.25 ounces
Distress or Rescue Flower Remedy	4 droppers
Lavender	10 drops
Chamomile, Roman	8 drops
Patchouli	7 drops

Instructions: In a 4 ounce bottle, combine essential oils and Distress or Rescue Remedy. Mix well. Next, add in the aqua-sol silver and liquid plant enzymes. Shake well.

Directions for Use: Apply to affected areas as needed to relieve itching, redness, inflammation and dryness. Also good for burns, scrapes, sunburns and skin rashes.

Herbal Insect Repellent

Liquid Plant Enzymes	3.5 ounces
Unscented Carrier Oil	.50 ounces
Thyme	5 drops
Lavender	4 drops
Geranium	5 drops
Peppermint	5 drops
Cinnamon	5 drops
Citronella	5 drops

Instructions: In a 4 ounce bottle, combine the essential oils and carrier oil. Shake well. Add in the liquid plant enzymes and shake well.

Directions for Use: Apply to exposed skin surfaces five to ten minutes before going outside to repel mosquitoes and insects. Safe for babies.

Inflammation Relief Cream

Aloe Vera Gel	3 ounces
Arnica and/or Calendula Cream	.50 ounces
MSM Cream	.50 ounces
Yarrow	2 drops
Chamomile, Roman	10 drops
Lavender	8 drops
Peppermint	5 drops
Cypress	5 drops

Instructions: In a 4 ounce glass jar, mix the Arnica and/or Calendula Cream and MSM cream. Next, add in the essential oils and aloe vera gel and mix well.

Directions for Use: Apply to inflamed area hourly until inflammation and swelling is reduced. Repeat every three to four hours thereafter.

Insomniac Mist

Distilled Water	2 ounces
Distress or Rescue Flower Remedy	4 droppers
Lavender	8 drops
Chamomile, Roman	4 drops
Patchouli	4 drops
Myrrh	3 drops

Instructions: In a 2 ounce bottle, combine the essential oils and Distress or Rescue Remedy and mix well. Next, add in the distilled water. Shake well. For dehydrated and chronically ill persons, use liquid plant enzymes instead of water.

Directions for Use: Spray yourself three to four times and the surrounding area (bed linens, pajamas, blanket, etc.) after dinner, one hour before bed and at bedtime. Also use if you wake up in the middle of the night.

Intestinal Soother

Unscented Carrier Oil	.33 ounces
Chamomile, Roman	8 drops
Peppermint	2 drops
Lavender	1 drop
Marjoram	1 drop

Instructions: In a .33 ounce roll-on bottle, mix the essential oils and carrier oil. Shake well.

Directions for Use: Apply to abdomen area as needed for relief of intestinal cramping, bloating, indigestion and spasms. For best results, apply generously, wait five minutes and apply again.

Jock Itch Relief

Liquid Plant Enzymes	1.75 ounces
Arnica Oil	.25 ounces
Patchouli	6 drops
Roman Chamomile	5 drops
Tea Tree	4 drops
Bergamot	2 drops
Lavender	3 drops

Instructions: In a 2 ounce bottle, combine the essential oils and arnica oil. Shake well. Add in the liquid plant enzymes and shake well.

Directions for Use: Apply to affected area two to three times daily, and as needed for redness, itching and discomfort.

Labor Enhancing Set

Contract (stimulate)

Evening Primrose Oil	1 ounce
Rose	2 drops
Geranium	4 drops
Clary sage	4 drops

Relax (calm)

Progesterone Cream	.50 ounces
Aloe Vera Gel	.50 ounces
Lavender	2 drops
Marjoram	1 drop
Cinnamon	2 drops
Jasmine	2 drops

Instructions: **Contract** - In a 1oz. bottle, combine the essential oils and evening primrose oil. Shake well.

Relax - in a 1 oz. jar, combine the progesterone cream and essential oils. Mix well. Add in the aloe vera gel and mix well.

Directions for Use: During labor, your body will contract and relax in intervals. Using this 1-2 system will mimic your body's natural response to labor, support and enhance the body during this time. You will rotate use between these two blends. When contractions start, apply the contract blend to the uterus area, lower back and ankle bones (inside and out). Wait about 2-5 minutes and apply the relax blend in the same manner. This interval time will decrease as your contraction become closer together. You will repeat this process in sync with your contractions. As contractions increase in frequency, so will your use of these two formulas in a rotation manner. These blends are also helpful for post-partum depression, anxiety and nervousness that goes along with becoming a new parent.

Migraine Relief Stick

Unscented Carrier Oil	.33 ounces
Peppermint	4 drops
Eucalyptus	4 drops
Chamomile, Roman	3 drops
Helichrysum	1 drop

Instructions: In a .33 ounce roll-on bottle, combine the essential oils and unscented carrier oil. Mix well.

Directions for Use: Apply to temples, hairline, back of neck and bottoms of feet before or at the onset of a migraine headache. Rotate with ice packs every five to ten minutes.

Mold Buster Spray

Liquid Plant Enzymes	8 ounces
Cinnamon	9 drops
Oregano	9 drops
Patchouli	8 drops
Thyme	10 drops
Eucalyptus	9 drops
Tea Tree	10 drops

Instructions: In an 8 ounce bottle, combine the essential oils and liquid plant enzymes. Shake well.

Directions for Use: Apply to areas of mold, window sills, bathrooms, etc. Use at least once daily for acute situations and two to three times daily for more serious situations.

Mood Balance

Liquid Plant Enzymes	2 ounces
Distress or Rescue Flower Remedy	2 droppers
Geranium	8 drops
Frankincense	8 drops
Bergamot	4 drops

Instructions: In a 2 ounce bottle, combine the essential oils and Distress or Rescue Remedy. Mix well. Add in the liquid plant enzymes and shake well.

Directions for Use: Spray generously around you and take in a deep breath, smelling the balancing essential oils. Use as often as needed.

Nervous Pet Relief

Liquid Plant Enzymes	2 ounces
Distress or Rescue Flower Remedy	2 droppers
Crab Apple Flower Essence (optional)	4 drops
Roman Chamomile	3 drops
Lavender	2 drops
Geranium	1 drop
Red Mandarin	3 drops
Sandalwood	1 drop

Instructions: In a 2 ounce bottle, combine the essential oils and both Flower Remedies. Mix well. Add in the liquid plant enzymes and shake well.

Directions for Use: Apply to surrounding area around pet, or on a bandana around their neck to calm nervous conditions. Use as needed.

PMS Abdomen Rub

Unscented Carrier Oil	.33 ounces
Lavender	2 drops
Chamomile, Roman	1 drop
Geranium	3 drops
Clary Sage	2 drops
Spearmint	3 drops
Basil, sweet	1 drop

Instructions: In a .33 ounce roll-on bottle, combine the essential oils and unscented massage oil. Shake well.

Directions for Use: Apply to abdomen area to relieve cramps associated with PMS. Also relieves mood swings, irritability and hot flashes when applied to temples, under nose and wrists.

Pneumonia

Aloe Vera Gel	75 ounces
Golden Salve	.25 ounces
Unscented Lotion or Carrier Oil	1 ounce
Inula	6 drops
Ammi visnaga	5 drops
Ravinsara	6 drops

Instructions: In a 2 ounce jar, mix the golden salve and aloe vera gel until a smooth consistency. Next, add the essential oils and blend. Last, add the unscented lotion or oil and mix well.

Directions for Use: Apply to chest, back (between shoulder blades), sinus areas on the face and to the bottom of the feet three to four times daily.

Respiratory Congestion (dry cough and congestion)

Aloe Vera Gel	1 ounce
Unscented Carrier Oil	1 ounce
Rosemary	4 drops
Eucalyptus	5 drops
Pine	2 drops
Sandalwood	4 drops
Myrrh	3 drops

Instructions: In a 2 ounce jar, combine the essential oils with the aloe vera gel and unscented carrier oil. Mix well.

Directions for Use: Apply to the chest area and middle of back (between the shoulder blades). This will help support the lungs from both sides of the body. Also, apply to the bottoms of your feet. Use at least twice daily.

Ringworm and Roundworms

Liquid Plant Enzymes	4 ounces
Eucalyptus	6 drops
Chamomile, Roman	2 drops
Cinnamon	5 drops
Thyme, Sweet	6 drops
Clove	5 drops
Oregano	5 drops

Instructions: In a 4 ounce bottle, combine the essential oils and liquid plant enzymes. Shake well.

Directions for Use: Spray affected area, clothes and bed linens three to four times daily.

Romance Perfume

Unscented Carrier Oil	.33 ounces
Ylang Ylang	5 drops
Neroli	3 drops
Jasmine	2 drops
Cinnamon	1 drop

Instructions: In a .33 ounce glass roll-on bottle, add in half of the carrier oil with the essential oils. Mix well, then add in the remaining carrier oil. Shake well.

Directions for Use: Apply to temples, neck, wrist and other pulse points to release this sensual fragrance. Also, apply to the tips of the hair for a longer lasting scent.

Sciatica Mist

Liquid Plant Enzymes	4 ounces
Helichrysum	8 drops
Marjoram	8 drops
Lavender	10 drops
Rose	6 drops

Instructions: In a 4 ounce bottle, combine the essential oils and liquid plant enzymes. Shake well.

Directions for Use: Spray every 15-60 minutes to sciatic area or as needed for pain relief. On a maintenance basis, spray three to four times daily. Let the spray soak in on its own.

Shaving Gel for Men

Castile Soap	3 ounces
Aloe Vera Gel	1 ounce
Tea Tree	8 drops
Lavender	14 drops
Spearmint	5 drops

Instructions: In a 4 ounce bottle, combine the essential oils, aloe vera gel and castile soap, respectively. Shake well.

Directions for Use: Apply to damp face before shaving. Offers a clean, close, refreshing shave without creating nicks and cuts and extends the life of your razor.

Shave Gel for Women

Castile Soap	3 ounces
Aloe Vera Gel	1 ounce
Lavender	12 drops
Chamomile	5 drops
Patchouli	5 drops
Mandarin, Red	4 drops

Instructions: In a 4 ounce bottle, combine the essential oils, aloe vera gel and castile soap, respectively. Shake well.

Directions for Use: Apply to damp skin before shaving. It moisturizes and hydrates the skin while offering a clean, close, refreshing shave without creating nicks and cuts and extends the life of your razor.

Shingle Relief Spray

Liquid Plant Enzymes	2 ounces
Aqua-sol Silver	1 dropper
Bergamot	5 drops
Lavender	6 drops
Chamomile, Roman	3 drops
Frankincense	3 drops
Thyme	2 drops

Instructions: In a 2 ounce bottle, combine the essential oils, aqua-sol silver and liquid plant enzymes, respectively. Shake well.

Directions for Use: Apply to affected area at least three times daily and as needed for itching, inflammation, pain and discomfort.

Skin Irritations

Unscented Lotion	1 ounce
Aloe Vera Gel	.50 ounces
Pau D'Arco Lotion	.50 ounces
Patchouli	4 drops
Myrrh	4 drops
Chamomile, Roman	4 drops
Lavender	3 drops
Bergamot	3 drops
Helichrysum	2 drops

Instructions: In a 2 ounce jar, mix the aloe vera gel and pau d' arco lotion with the essential oils. Next, add in the unscented lotion and mix well.

Directions for Use: Apply to affected area at least three times daily and as needed for itching, inflammation, dryness, cracked and chapped skin.

Sports Rub

MSM Cream	.50 ounces
Arnica and/or Calendula Cream	.50 ounces
Unscented Lotion	1 ounce
Cypress	5 drops
Black Pepper	4 drops
Lavender	4 drops
Chamomile, Roman	5 drops
Helichrysum	2 drops

Instructions: In a 2 ounce jar, mix the MSM Cream, and Arnica and/or Calendula Cream. Next, add in the essential oils and unscented lotion. Mix well until all essential oils and carriers are blended.

Directions for Use: Apply two to three times daily to muscles, ligaments, tendons and joints to relieve swelling, inflammations, pain, sprains, pulls and overuse.

Stop Smoking

Unscented Carrier Oil	.33 ounces
Melissa	3 drops
Bergamot	4 drops
Clary sage	3 drops
Helichrysum	1 drop

Instructions: In a .33 ounce roll-on bottle, combine the essential oils and unscented massage oil.   Shake well.

Directions for Use: Use as often as needed to calm and reduce cravings for nicotine. Inhale the scents and/or apply to the skin around the nose area, wrists and other pulse points.

Study Buddy

Unscented Carrier Oil	.33 ounces
Rosemary	2 drops
Peppermint	3 drops
Lemon	3 drops
Mandarin, Red	2 drops

Instructions: In a .33 ounce roll-on bottle, combine the essential oils and unscented massage oil. Shake well.

Directions for Use: Apply to wrists, neck, temples and other pulse points when studying, taking a test or in need of concentration, focus and alertness. For memory recall, smell this blend when you are studying and when you are retrieving the information.

Stress Away

Aloe Vera Gel	15 ml
Distress or Rescue Flower Remedy	4 drops
Bergamot	3 drops
Lavender	2 drops
Mandarin, Red	2 drops

Instructions: In a 15 ml amber bottle, combine the essential oils, Distress or Rescue Remedy and aloe vera gel. Shake well.

Directions for Use: Apply to wrists, hands, neck, face and other pulse points as needed to calm stress and quiet the mind. Also, great to reduce anxiety and nervousness.

Stress Relief Spray

Liquid Plant Enzymes	2 ounces
Distress or Rescue Flower Remedy	2 droppers
Cinnamon	5 drops
Clove	3 drops
Mandarin	5 drops
Lemon	4 drops
Pine	2 drops

Instructions: In a 2 ounce bottle, combine the essential oils and Distress or Rescue Remedy. Mix well. Then add in the liquid plant enzymes. Shake well.

Directions for Use: Spray around you three to four times while taking in a deep breath. Use at least three times daily and as needed to relieve stressful events and situations.

Submissive Urination for Pets

Liquid Plant Enzymes	2 ounces
Distress or Rescue Flower Remedy	2 droppers
Frankincense	4 drops
Lavender	4 drops
Juniper	2 drops
Pine	1 drop

Instructions: In a 2 ounce bottle, combine the essential oils and the Distress or Rescue Remedy. Mix well. Then add in the liquid plant enzymes and shake well.

Directions for Use: Spray 2-3 times around the pet before and during times of submissive urination situations. Herbally, you may want to consider adding in Cornsilk to their diet. Emotionally, it has been linked to fear of a male figure.

Sunburn Soother

Vitamin E Oil	1 Tablespoon
Jojoba Oil	1 Tablespoon
Aqua-sol Silver	.25 ounces
Aloe Vera Gel	.50 ounces
Liquid Plant Enzymes	1.25 ounces
Distress or Rescue Flower Remedy	2 droppers
Peppermint	3 drops
Lavender	10 drops
Tea tree	4 drops
Helichrysum	2 drops

Instructions: In a 2 ounce bottle, combine the essential oils, jojoba oil, vitamin E oil, Distress or Rescue Remedy and aloe vera gel. Mix well. Next, add in the aqua-sol silver and liquid plant enzymes. Shake well.

Directions for Use: Spray sunburned area at least three to four times daily and as needed for itching, flaking skin, pain and discomfort.

Teething Roll-on

Extra Virgin Olive Oil	.50 ounces
Chamomile, Roman	6 drops

Instructions: In a .5 ounce bottle or jar, combine the essential oil in the olive oil. Mix well.

Directions for Use: Apply to clean fingertip and massage onto teething gums as needed for pain and discomfort. To reduce a teething induced fever, apply to temples, neck, jaw line and feet.

Thunderstorm Fright (for children and pets)

Liquid Plant Enzymes	2 ounces
Distress or Rescue Flower Remedy	4 droppers
Lavender	3 drops
Roman Chamomile	2 drops
Frankincense	3 drops
Jasmine	2 drops
Red Mandarin	2 drops

Instructions: In a 2 ounce bottle, combine the essential oils and the Distress or Rescue Remedy. Mix well. Then add in the liquid plant enzymes and shake well.

Directions for Use: Apply to surrounding area up to two hours before exposure to thunderstorm or fireworks. Lightly mist, with one to two sprays in air every 15 minutes leading up to the frightening event, and as needed, in a well ventilated area. Combine with Distress or Rescue Remedy, internally as instructed on the bottle.

Tummy Ease Roll-on

Unscented Carrier Oil	.33 ounces
Peppermint	5 drops
Thyme	2 drops
Ginger	3 drops
Roman Chamomile	2 drops

Instructions: In a .33 ounce glass roll-on bottle, add in half of the carrier oil with the essential oils. Mix well, then add in the remaining carrier oil. Shake well.

Directions for Use: Apply to abdomen area for tummy upset, gas, bloating, discomfort and constipation.

Urinary Tract Infection

Aloe Vera Gel	2 ounces
Frankincense	5 drops
Juniper	4 drops
Lemon	3 drops
Pine	3 drops

Instructions: In a 2 ounce bottle, combine the essential oils and aloe vera gel (can substitute with unscented massage oil). Shake well.

Directions for Use: Massage into bladder and kidney areas two to three times daily and as needed for pain and discomfort. If frequent urinary tract infections persist, look to resolve any fearful situations that might be present as we hold fear in the kidneys.

Warts Away

Black Ointment	.33 ounces
Activated Charcoal	1 capsule
Golden Salve	.33 ounces
Arnica and/or Calendula Cream	.33 ounces
Aqua-sol Silver	1 dropper
Carrot Seed	2 drops
Lavender	6 drops
Tea Tree	2 drops
Helichrysum	2 drops
Chamomile, Roman	4 drops
Patchouli	4 drops

Instructions: In a 1 ounce jar, mix the black ointment, activated charcoal and golden salve until smooth. Next add in the Arnica/Calendula Cream, followed by the aqua-sol silver and essential oils. Mix well.

Directions for Use: Apply to affected area 4-6 times daily. File wart down every three days. There may be black, white or clear seeds or liquid that ooze from the wart. Protect it from getting infected.

Yeast Infection

Golden Salve	1 ounce
Lavender	3 drops
Chamomile, Roman	3 drops
Geranium	2 drops
Tea Tree	2 drops

Instructions: In a 1 ounce jar, soften the golden salve by stirring until smooth. Add in the essential oils and mix well.

Directions for Use: Apply to affected area twice daily and as needed to relieve pain, burning and discomfort. Can use for any fungal infection or skin irritation.

Therapeutic Properties Descriptions

Here are definitions for the properties listed for each essential oil and carrier profile. I've listed some of my favorite examples, but not limited to this list.

Analgesic: Relieves pain. Bay laurel, birch, eucalyptus, ginger, lavender, clove, marjoram and spearmint.

Antibacterial: Combats, destroys or suppresses bacteria. All essential oils are antibacterial, just in varying potencies.

Antidepressant: Combats depression, sadness and loss of interest. Bergamot, clary sage, melissa, neroli, sandalwood and St. John's Wort.

Anti-emetic: Calms, suppresses and reduces nausea and vomiting. Cardamom, chamomile (Roman), ginger, lemongrass, peppermint and spearmint.

Antifungal: Combats, destroys or suppresses fungus and mold. Lemon, oregano, patchouli, thyme and tea tree.

Antigalactagogue: Dries up breast milk. Birch, clary sage, parsley, peppermint, sage and spearmint.

Anti-inflammatory (Antiphlogistic): Combats or reduces inflammation. Chamomiles, fir oils, frankincense, ginger, helichrysum, myrrh, lavender, rose and yarrow.

Antioxidant: Combats oxidation such as free radical damage and "aging" of cells. All essential oils are antibacterial, just in varying potencies.

Antiparasitic: Combats, destroys or expels parasites. Clove, ginger, *Juniperus virginiana*, oakmoss, oregano, patchouli and tea tree.

Antispasmodic: Relieves spasms and cramping. Ammi visnaga, cardamom, chamomiles, ginger, peppermint, marjoram, neroli, and *Tanacetum annuum*.

Antiviral: Combats or destroys viruses. Ammi visnaga, bergamot, cinnamon, eucalyptus, lemon, lime and ravinsara.

Aphrodisiac: Arouses sexual desire. Cinnamon, geranium, jasmine, neroli, rose, sandalwood and ylang ylang.

Astringent: Contracts, tightens or tones body tissue and skin. Bergamot, cedar, geranium, lemongrass, rosemary and thyme.

Cardiotonic: Strengthens or tones the heart and circulatory system. Grapefruit, orange, rose, spikenard, turmeric and ylang ylang.

Carminative: Aids in the expulsion of gas from the intestines. Anise, chamomile, ginger, lemon, peppermint and thyme.

Cephalic: Relating to the head and brain. Basil, Cedar (atlas), clary sage, jasmine, lemon, lemongrass, peppermint and rosemary.

Cholagogue: Aids in the elimination of bile from the gall bladder and bile ducts. Chamomile, grapefruit, helichrysum, lavender, ledum, oregano, peppermint and turmeric.

Choleretic: Increases or stimulates bile production from the liver. Helichrysum, orange, rose, rosemary and sage.

Cicatrisant: Promotes healing through the formation of scar tissue. Carrot seed, helichrysum, mandarin, frankincense, patchouli and yarrow.

Cytophylactic: Encourages new cell growth or cellular regeneration. Frankincense, helichrysum, palmarosa, patchouli and turmeric.

Decongestant: Relieves or releases nasal congestion and other body fluids. Eucalyptus, inula, frankincense, lemon, peppermint, rosemary and thyme.

Demulcent: Mucilaginous; relieves and soothes inflamed and irritated mucosal membranes. Fenugreek, myrrh, oakmoss, sandalwood and violet.

Deodorant: Eliminates or combats body odors. Sage, coriander, bergamot, clary sage, lemon and thyme.

Depurative: Assists in the purification and detoxification process. Cilantro, coriander, grapefruit, orris root, sage and turmeric.

Diaphoretic: Induces and increases perspiration. Basil, cinnamon, clove, eucalyptus, ginger, oregano and tea tree.

Digestive: Assisting and supporting the digestive function. Basil (holy), chamomiles, fennel, ginger, peppermint and turmeric.

Diuretic: Helps promote fluid elimination via kidneys and urine. Celery seed, cypress, geranium, grapefruit, juniper, may chang and sandalwood.

Emetic: Induces and causes vomiting. Angelica, orris root and birch.

Emmenagogue: Stimulates reproductive blood blow and promotes menstruation. Clary sage, geranium, jasmine, juniper, and neroli rosemary.

Expectorant: Encourages the breakup of and promotes the expulsion of mucus. Chamomile, eucalyptus, oregano, pine, peppermint, myrrh and sandalwood.

Febrifuge: Reduces fever or excess heat. Bergamot, chamomile, lemon, parsley, peppermint, rose and vetiver.

Galactagogue: Encourages or promotes the production of breast milk. Fenugreek, jasmine, fennel and lemongrass.

Hepatic: Relating or associated with the liver. Carrot seed, chamomiles, cypress, helichrysum lemon, monarda and rose.

Hepatotoxic: Can cause liver toxicity in high amounts, especially when ingested. Anise, clove, pennyroyal, tarragon, thuja and wintergreen.

Homeostatic: A state of equilibrium and internal stability maintained by self-regulating biological and metabolic processes of the mind and body. It is a state of perfect balance, harmony and well-being. David Stewart in his *The Chemistry of Essential oils Made Simple* book stated it best, "Essential oils possess homeostatic intelligence", so all essential oils are homeostatic.

Hypertensive: Increases blood pressure. Eucalyptus, oregano, rosemary, sage and thyme.

Hypotensive: Reduces blood pressure. Chamomile, citrus, clary sage, lavender, marjoram, rose and ylang ylang.

Insecticide: Combats and repels insects. Anise, citronella, eucalyptus, niaouli, patchouli, peppermint and thyme.

Mucolytic: Breaks down and reduces the viscosity of mucus. Basil, benzoin, frankincense, galbanum, inula, myrrh, rosemary and sandalwood.

Nervine: Supports the nervous system and nerves. Basil, bay laurel, clary sage, helichrysum, lavender, marjoram and ravinsara.

Nutritive: Provides nourishment. Carrot seed, cardamom, orange, turmeric and yuzu.

Purgative: Produces movement, purging or cleaning of the bowels. Chamomiles, fennel, ginger, peppermint, orris root and thyme.

Relaxant: Calms or relaxes the nerves, organs, body and mind. Chamomiles, frankincense, lavender, mandarin, marjoram, sage, neroli and ylang ylang.

Rubefacient: Increases redness of the skin via vasodilation and circulation. Bergamot, cypress, carrot, frankincense, lavender, pine, rosemary and spruce.

Sedative: Induces and inspires sedation to quiet irritability and over-excitement. Chamomiles, clary sage, davana, hyssop, jasmine, lavender marjoram and spikenard.

Stimulant: Enhances and increases circulation, movements of body and mind. Black pepper, cinnamon, cypress, eucalyptus and rosemary.

Stomachic: Assists digestion, promotes appetite or stimulates the stomach function. Basil, bergamot, chamomile, fennel, ginger, peppermint, spearmint and turmeric.

Styptic: Arrest bleeding. Benzoin, goldenrod, jasmine, spruce and yarrow.

Sudorific: Induces sweating. Basil, cinnamon, juniper, eucalyptus, ginger, rosemary, sandalwood and tea tree.

Vasoconstrictor: Constricts or tightens the blood vessels. Benzoin, chamomile, cypress, lavender, marjoram, peppermint, rose and ylang ylang.

Vasodilative: Opens the blood vessels. Eucalyptus, oregano, rosemary, sage and thyme.

Vermifuge: Destroys or expels worms. Cinnamon, clove, niaouli, oregano, patchouli and savory.

Vulnerary: Wound healing. Chamomile, frankincense, helichrysum, lavender, myrrh, and tea tree.

Bibliography

Book References

Balas, Kimberly N.D. (2002). Applied Aromatherapy. Tree of Light Publishing.

Battaglia, Salvatore. (1995) *The Complete Guide To Aromatherapy*. The Perfect Potion.

Berkowsky, Dr. Bruce. (2003-2015) *Spiritual PhytoEssencing Materia Medica*. www.NaturalHealthScience.com; (2010) *Six Element Paradigm Workbook*

Buckle, Jane Ph.D., RN. (2015, 2003, 1997) C*linical Aromatherapy: Essential oils in Healthcare*

Clarke, Sue. (2002) *Essential Chemistry for Safe Aromatherapy*

Djilani, Abdelouaheb & Dicko, Amadou. (2012) The Therapeutic Benefits of Essential Oils, Nutrition, Well-Being and Health, Dr. Jaouad Bouayed (Ed.), ISBN: 978-953-51-0125-3, InTech, Available from: http://www.intechopen.com/books/nutrition-well-being-and-health/the-therapeutic-benefits-of-essential-oils

Gershon, Michael D., Ph.D. (1998) *The Second Brain: The Scientific Basis of Gut Instinct and a Groundbreaking New Understanding of Nervous Disorders of the Stomach and Intestines*

Gonzales, Maria-Dolores. Feb. 2004. CNHP Clinical Aromatherapy Seminar

Jones, Larissa. (2001-02) *Aromatherapy For Body, Mind & Spirit*. Evergreen Aromatherapy.

Hay, Louise L. (1982) *Heal Your Body*

Herb Allure. (2004) *Hart Aromatherapy*. www.herballure.com

Hochell Pressimone, Jennifer. (2005) *JennScents Aromatherapy Custom Blending Bar Business Guide*. JennScents, Inc. www.JennScents.com, www.JennScentsInstitute.com; *Aromatherapy Spiritual PhytoEssencing: Deep Emotional, Body, Mind, Spirit & Soul Healing Seminar*, Jennifer Hochell Pressimone, Aug 2014, NAHA WOA VII

Horne, Steven. (2002-2005) *Various Classes and Seminars*. Tree of Light Publishing. www.treelite.com; (2006) *Traditional Chinese Medicine: Eastern Remedies for Western Ailments;* (2003) *The Comprehensive Guide to Nature's Sunshine Products*. Tree of Light Publishing. www.treelite.com

Kaminski, Patricia and Katz, Richard. (2004) *Flower Essence Repertory*

Mercola, Joseph M.D. (various articles) http://www.mercola.com/

Mojay, Gabriel. (2000) *Aromatherapy for Healing the Spirit*

National Association of Holistic Aromatherapy, www.NAHA.org

Pålsson K, Jaenson TG, Baeckström P, Borg-Karlson AK. (January 2008). "Tick repellent substances in the essential oil of Tanacetum vulgare". Journal of

Medical Entomology 45 (1): 88–93. doi:10.1603/0022-2585(2008)45[88:TRSITE]2.0.CO;2. PMID 18283947

Pert, Candace B., Ph.D. (1997) *Molecules of Emotion*

Pub Med. (various published scientific and research studies) www.PubMed.com

Rose, Jeanne. (1992) *The Aromatherapy Book*. Herbal Studies Course/Jeanne Rose; (2000) *Herbal Body Book, The Herbal Way To Natural Beauty & Health For Men & Women*. Frog, Ltd.; (1999) *375 Essential Oils And Hydrosols*. Frog, Ltd.; http://www.encognitive.com/node/14717

Sherman, Denise. (2002) *Aromatherapy Basic Training*. Vintage Essentials

Stewart, David. (2006) The Chemistry of Essential Oils Made Simple

Tisserand, Robert. (2002) *Essential Oil Safety: A Guide for Health Care Professionals*

Zukav, Gary & Francis, Linda (2001) *The Heart of the Soul: Emotional Awareness*

Reference Charts

Essential Oils for Physical Concerns

✓ Digestion

Gas, bloating, indigestion	Basil, cardamom, chamomiles, fennel, ginger, mints, thyme, yuzu
Hiatal hernia	Chamomiles, fennel, ginger, lemon, marjoram, turmeric
Nausea	Chamomile (Roman), ginger, lemon, lemongrass, peppermint, spearmint
Reflux, Acid & Silent	Cardamom, ginger, lemon, nutmeg
Toothache	Birch, clove, myrrh, sandalwood

✓ Intestinal

Constipation	Basil, cedar, myrrh, oakmoss, patchouli, rosemary
Diarrhea	Chamomile, lemongrass, marjoram, nutmeg, St. John's Wort, turmeric
H. Pylori	Balsam peru, clove, inula, oregano, savory
Hemorrhoids	Chamomiles, cypress, frankincense, geranium, lavender, turmeric, yarrow
IBS, Leaky Gut	Chamomiles, ginger, lemon, mints, marjoram, yarrow
Intestinal Parasites	Cinnamon, clove, ginger, oregano, patchouli, tea tree

✓ Immune

	All Essential Oils
Allergies	Eucalyptus, frankincense, lavender, lemongrass, mints, turmeric
Fever	Chamomiles, citrus, ginger, lavender, lemongrass, mints, parsley, turmeric
Platelets, Increase	Carrot seed, ginger, lemon, mints, neroli, orange, rosemary, yarrow
Viral (cold sores, shingles)	Ammi visnaga, bergamot, cinnamon, clove, lemon, lemongrass, melissa, oregano, palmarosa, thyme, yarrow
WBC, Increase	Catnip, lemon, lemongrass, niaouli

Respiratory

Bronchitis	Ammi visnaga, cedar, clove, elemi, eucalyptus, inula, pine, ravinsara, sandalwood, thyme
Cough, Dry	Balsam peru, basil, benzoin, frankincense, pine, sandalwood, tarragon, vetiver
Cough, Wet	Anise, blue cypress, cedar, citronella, eucalyptus, parsley, patchouli, tea tree
Earaches	Cajeput, lemon, helichrysum, oregano
Sinus Issues	Eucalyptus, firs, myrtle, niaouli, thyme, tea tree, wintergreen
Sore Throat	Bergamot, frankincense, lavender, lemon, myrrh, sage, sandalwood, thyme

Nervous

Anxiety; Nervous	Cinnamon, citrus, clary sage, jasmine, lavender, neroli, St. John's Wort, yuzu
Nerve Pain	Basil, bay laurel, birch, clary sage, clove, marjoram, wintergreen

Glandular

Adrenal	Chamomile, orange, pine, *Tanacetum annuum*, vetiver, yarrow
Hepatic (liver)	Chamomile, helichrysum, lemon, rose
Men, Hormone Balance	Cilantro, cinnamon, lavender, rose, spruce, vetiver, ylang ylang
Pancreas, Blood Sugar	Cinnamon, coriander, fennel, grapefruit, parsley, spruce, thyme
Thyroid, Support	Celery seed, davana, geranium, melissa, myrrh, myrtle, pine, *Tanacetum annuum*
Thyroid, Boost	Black pepper, geranium, fir, myrrh, myrtle, orange, palmarosa, rosemary
Women, Hormone Balance (PMS, Menopause)	Angelica, carrot seed, chamomile, citrus, clary sage, geranium, ginger, lemon, mints, pine, sandalwood, vetiver, yarrow

Urinary

Bedwetting	Frankincense, geranium, lavender
Bladder/Kidney Weakness	Carrot, fennel, frankincense, oregano, rosewood, sandalwood; St. John's Wort
Bladder, Overactive	Ammi visnaga, fennel, fir (douglas), goldenrod, oregano, sandalwood
Edema/Water Retention; Cleansing	Cypress, grapefruit, juniper, lemon, patchouli, pine
Gout	Angelica, cinnamon, celery seed, citrus, juniper, petitgrain, rosemary
Kidney Stones	Cedar (Virg.), chamomiles, geranium, goldenrod, eucalyptus, niaouli, palo santo, rosemary

Circulatory

Blood Pressure, high	Helichrysum, lemon, peppermint, rose, ylang ylang
Blood Pressure, low	Oregano, rosemary, thyme
Brain, cephalic	Basil, cedar atlas, citrus, jasmine, lemon, mints, rosemary
Heart Palpitations	Rose, ylang ylang
Lymphatic Congestion	Cypress, geranium, grapefruit, lemon, patchouli
Poor Circulation; Vein health	Basil, black pepper, citrus, cypress, ginger, oregano, rose, rosemary, thyme, yarrow, yuzu

Structural

	(Hair, nails and skin)
Alopecia (hair loss)	Angelica, black pepper, clary sage, rosemary, sage, ylang ylang
Arthritis; Rheumatism	Basil, black pepper, firs, frankincense, ginger, ho leaf, juniper, may chang, ravinsara, turmeric
Backache, pain	Birch, clary sage, clove, frankincense, ginger, marjoram, rosemary, spikenard, turmeric
Bone Strength	Frankincense, geranium, lavender, myrrh, oregano, rosemary, thyme
Fibromyalgia/Chronic Fatigue	Black pepper, cinnamon, clary sage, ho leaf, ravinsara, St. John's Wort, turmeric, vetiver

Structural Con't.

Mobility, Flexibility	Angelica, bay laurel, cajeput, cedar, eucalyptus, frankincense, ginger, turmeric
Muscle & Joint Pain, Sprain; Stiffness	Black pepper, clove, frankincense, lemongrass, marjoram, rose, turmeric
Muscle Spasms	Bay laurel, chamomiles, clary sage, lavender, marjoram, oregano, neroli
Skin, Irritations (acne, eczema, psoriasis, rash)	Bergamot, helichrysum, geranium, lavender, patchouli, yarrow
Skin Itching, insect bites	Bergamot, chamomiles, frankincense, lavender, ledum, oakmoss, patchouli
Skin Scarring, pigmentation	Carrot, frankincense, helichrysum, lavender, myrrh, patchouli, rose

Essential Oils for Mental Concerns

Digestion

Depression	Basil, citrus, clary sage, frankincense, geranium, helichrysum, jasmine, lemongrass, may chang, rose
Confusion	Ammi visnaga, camphor, citrus, cypress, geranium, jasmine, mints, patchouli, rosemary, sandalwood
Indecisive	Black pepper, cypress, firs, frankincense, geranium, juniper, orange, patchouli, sandalwood, spikenard
Negative Thoughts	Angelica, basil, bay laurel, cedar, citrus, geranium, lemongrass, peppermint, pine, sage, tea tree

Intestinal

Distracted easily	Balsam peru, citronella, eucalyptus, lemon, myrtle, orange, palmarosa, rose, rosemary, vetiver
Mental Chatter; Racing Thoughts	Benzoin, chamomiles, clary sage, eucalyptus, firs, inula, lavender, myrrh, *Tanacetum annuum*, yuzu
Over-thinking	Basil, benzoin, cardamom, chamomiles, fennel, frankincense, marjoram, myrrh, orange, ylang ylang

Immune

All Essential Oils	
Creative thinking	Angelica, bay laurel, citrus, cinnamon, clary sage, lemongrass, nutmeg, orange, violet
Inspiration	Bay laurel, clary sage, clove, lemon, lemongrass, mints, orris root, rosemary, spikenard
Learning Ability	Cedar (atlas), cilantro, frankincense, lavender, lemon, rosemary, sage, vetiver
Positive; Optimistic	Angelica, citrus, clary sage, myrtle, pine, ravinsara, rose, spruce, vanilla, ylang ylang

Respiratory

Problem solving	Basil, birch, cedar, cypress, eucalyptus, inula, lemon, orange, niaouli, rosemary, sage, vetiver
Stutter; Speech	Cedar (atlas), eucalyptus, lemon, mints, neroli, orange, rosemary, sandalwood, vetiver

Nervous

Addictions	Basil, bergamot, clary sage, coriander, fennel, firs, geranium, helichrysum, lemon, melissa, sandalwood
Insomnia	Chamomiles, cistus, fennel, frankincense, geranium, lavender, patchouli, sandalwood
Stress	All essential oils

Glandular

Anxiety	Bergamot, chamomile, cedar, cinnamon, geranium, jasmine, lavender, neroli, pine, ylang ylang, yuzu
Judgmental	Basil, bergamot, lemongrass, lime, orange, orris root, petitgrain, pine, patchouli, rosewood, turmeric
Lethargy	Birch, cardamom, carrot seed, clove, orris root, pine, ravinsara, spearmint, tarragon, tea tree
Panic attack	Bergamot, clary sage, cinnamon, grapefruit, inula, marjoram, melissa, ravinsara, spruce, ylang ylang

Urinary

Articulate communication	Angelica, blue cypress, jasmine, lemon, myrrh, orris root, peppermint, rosemary
Determination	Bay laurel, blue cypress, dill, elemi, goldenrod, myrrh, palo santo, tarragon, turmeric
Fear of public speaking; agoraphobia	Balsam peru, bay laurel, cinnamon, clary sage, galbanum, frankincense, orange, savory, vetiver

Circulatory

Concentration	Basil, bay laurel, black pepper, cedar, firs, inula, juniper, lemon, lemongrass, rosemary, thyme
Focus	Birch, blue cypress, eucalyptus, lemon, mints, orange, niaouli, rosemary, tea tree
Mental clarity	Basil, cedar, fennel, jasmine, lemon, lemongrass, may chang, mints, niaouli, rosemary, vetiver
Mental fatigue	Ammi visnaga, cardamom, citrus, eucalyptus, mints, pine, ravinsara, rosemary, vetiver

Structural (Hair, nails and skin)

Cognitive Functions	Anise, basil, black pepper, cedar, frankincense, mints, rosemary, vetiver, turmeric
Confidence	Bay laurel, black pepper, clary sage, firs, mints, rosemary, *Tanacetum annuum*, vetiver, ylang ylang
Headaches, general	Basil, frankincense, ginger, grapefruit, lavender, lemongrass, peppermint, turmeric
Headaches, hormone	Frankincense, geranium, helichrysum, jasmine, lemongrass, peppermint, pine, sandalwood
Headaches, vasoconstrictive	Basil, black pepper, coriander, eucalyptus, ginger, frankincense, lavender, mints, rosemary
Headaches, vasodilative	Chamomile, helichrysum, lemon, lime, marjoram, may chang, peppermint, vetiver, ylang ylang

Essential Oils for Emotional Concerns

Digestion	
Digest/Accept a situation	Benzoin, chamomiles, black pepper, fennel, melissa, peppermint, ravinsara, sandalwood, ylang ylang
Hopeless; Despair	Blue cypress, catnip, cilantro, cinnamon, frankincense, helichrysum, lemon, lemongrass, orris root, pine, spikenard
Self-esteem	Bay laurel, cinnamon, eucalyptus, geranium, jasmine, lemongrass, monarda, palmarosa, spearmint
Suppression	Cinnamon, dill, eucalyptus, grapefruit, mints orange, rosemary, thyme, yuzu
Worthiness	Basil, black pepper, cypress, eucalyptus, geranium, mints, tarragon, turmeric, vetiver, yarrow

Intestinal	
Negative	Angelica, cedar, cilantro, citrus, firs, geranium, juniper, lemongrass, lime, myrrh, palo santo, sage
Worry	Basil, chamomiles, geranium, grapefruit, lavender, myrrh, niaouli, rosemary, sandalwood, vetiver
Withdrawn	Chamomiles, clary sage, cajeput, juniper, lemon, mints, oregano, savory, rosemary, yuzu

Immune	All Essential Oils
Attacked, feelings of	Basil, citronella, davana, fennel, oregano, patchouli, *Tanacetum annuum*, tarragon, tea tree
Invasion of space and boundaries	Clove, grapefruit, eucalyptus, juniper, ledum, nutmeg, *Tanacetum annuum*, spearmint, tea tree
Lack of purpose	Balsam peru, blue cypress, cedar eucalyptus, monarda, myrrh, thyme, vetiver, ylang ylang
Overwhelmed; Overburdened	Basil, catnip, eucalyptus, firs, frankincense, inula, juniper, lemon, myrtle, rosemary, tea tree, yuzu
Self-doubt	Basil, citronella, cypress, firs, grapefruit, lemon, may chang, oregano, peppermint, spruce

Respiratory	
Abandonment	Bay laurel, chamomile, cinnamon, frankincense, may chang, nutmeg, palo santo, rosewood, vetiver
Grief	Bergamot, cinnamon, eucalyptus, geranium, marjoram, orange, ravinsara, rose, sandalwood, yarrow
Suffocated	Ammi visnaga, cajeput, eucalyptus, frankincense, lemon, myrrh, pine, ravinsara, thyme

Nervous	
Panic, Shock, Trauma	Ammi visnaga, clary sage, frankincense, geranium, orange, palmarosa, palo santo, pine, rose, yuzu
PTSD	Angelica, citrus, cinnamon, davana, nutmeg, palmarosa, rose, sandalwood, St. John's Wort, turmeric, vetiver

Glandular	
Anger; Rage	Chamomiles, helichrysum, lemon, peppermint, rose, vanilla, vetiver, ylang ylang

229

Glandular Con't.

Bitterness	Cinnamon, cypress, grapefruit, orange, palmarosa, patchouli, peppermint, sandalwood, rose, rosemary
Forgiveness	Angelica, davana, hyssop, grapefruit, lavender, monarda, parsley, patchouli, pine, rose, yuzu
Frustration; Irritability	Chamomiles, all citrus, frankincense, lemon, mints, petitgrain, pine, rose, ylang ylang
Jealous	Bergamot, chamomiles, cinnamon, davana, frankincense, grapefruit, orris root, vetiver, ylang ylang
Mood swings	Citrus, clary sage, firs, geranium, jasmine, palo santo, patchouli, sandalwood, St. John's Wort
Resentment	Ammi visnaga, black pepper, grapefruit, lemon, neroli, nutmeg, petitgrain, rose, spearmint

Urinary

Fear	Cinnamon, frankincense, juniper, niaouli, orange, palmarosa, pine, tarragon, ylang ylang
Guilt	Clary sage, frankincense, jasmine, niaouli, pine, ravinsara, ylang ylang
Shame	Cinnamon, eucalyptus, frankincense, geranium, grapefruit, juniper, lemon, orange, pine

Circulatory

Betrayal	Ammi visnaga, davana, lavender, ledum, palo santo, patchouli, rose, rosemary, vetiver
Broken heart	Bergamot, black pepper, helichrysum, marjoram, orange, rose, sandalwood, vanilla, ylang ylang
Emotionally cold	Anise, basil, cistus, oregano, rosemary, thyme
Loneliness, feel isolated	Bay laurel, benzoin, black pepper, carrot seed, clary sage, lemongrass, melissa, neroli, rosemary
Love	Angelica, bay laurel, chamomile, carrot seed, clary sage, jasmine, rose, rosemary, ylang ylang
Rejection	Bay laurel, cypress, lavender, lemon, melissa, orange, petitgrain, rose, vanilla, yarrow
Stuck emotions	Basil, carrot seed, citrus, cypress, grapefruit, inula, lavender, patchouli, pine, rosemary, sage, violet

Structural (Hair, nails and skin)

Courage (conquer)	Basil, bay laurel, cedars, cistus, davana, dill, fennel, frankincense, ginger, mints, orris root, thyme
Deep emotional wounds and pain	Ammi visnaga, balsam peru, benzoin, blue cypress, clary sage, davana, elemi, inula, ravinsara, yarrow
Defeated, feelings of	Bay laurel, bergamot, birch, cinnamon, firs, ho leaf, orange, ravinsara, tarragon, tea tree, violet
Disappointment	Cardamom, citrus, clary sage, davana, ginger, lemongrass, monarda, neroli, nutmeg, turmeric
Inner strength	Cardamom, cedars, cinnamon, cypress, davana, fennel, monarda, neroli, oregano, pine, yuzu
Self-defeating behaviors	Bergamot, cinnamon, geranium, lemon, orange, oregano, niaouli, ravinsara, tarragon, thyme, violet
Weakness, general emotions	Cardamom, cinnamon, eucalyptus, lemongrass, myrrh, niaouli, ravinsara, yarrow

General Index

232

233